STAYING BEAUTIFUL

COLOR PHOTOGRAPHY,
EXCEPT WHERE OTHERWISE CREDITED,
BY

NORMAN PARKINSON

BLACK-AND-WHITE PHOTOGRAPHY,
EXCEPT WHERE OTHERWISE CREDITED,
BY

EMERICK BRONSON

STAYING BEAUTIFUL

BEAUTY SECRETS AND ATTITUDES FROM
MY FORTY YEARS AS A MODEL

CARMEN
AND
ALFRED ALLAN LEWIS

HARPER & ROW, PUBLISHERS, New York
CAMBRIDGE, PHILADELPHIA, SAN FRANCISCO
LONDON, MEXICO CITY, SÃO PAULO, SINGAPORE, SYDNEY

1817

Undying gratitude to Beena Kamlani

Grateful acknowledgment is made for permission to reprint:

Photographs by Clifford Coffin, Horst, Irving Penn, Irwin Blumenfeld, John Rawlings, and Helmut Newton: Courtesy of *Vogue*. Copyright © 1946, 1947, 1948, 1951, and 1963 (renewed 1974, 1975, 1976, 1979) by The Condé Nast Publications Inc.

Photographs by Cecil Beaton: Courtesy Sotheby-Parke Bernet. *Vanity Fair photos:* Courtesy of Vanity Fair Mills, Inc.

A section of color photographs follows page 78

FIRST EDITION

Designer: Gloria Adelson/Lulu Graphics

Library of Congress Cataloging in Publication Data
Staying beautiful.
   1. Beauty, Personal. 2. Women—Health and hygiene.
3. Carmen. 4. Models, Fashion—United States—Biography.
I. Lewis, Alfred Allan. II. Title.
RA778.C2165 1985 646.7'042 84–48142
ISBN 0–06–015386–5

---

85 86 87 88 89 10 9 8 7 6 5 4 3 2 1

*To Papa
who's watching;
to Vincent
who said "You will
resume your career";
and to
"always there"
Zuggie and Crump*

CONTENTS

FIRST IMPRESSIONS

IT WAS DURING THE SUMMER of 1973, in East Hampton. We were having a dinner party and one of our guests, Margaret Leytess, called to ask if she might bring along somebody who was spending the weekend with her. When they arrived that evening, the stranger was introduced simply as "Carmen Kaplan." Her silver hair was pulled away from a face of such extraordinary beauty that one was literally stunned by it. She could have been any age—thirty, forty, fifty—but there was one thing of which I was certain: this Carmen was not remotely interested in the youth mania that was putting so many of my middle-aged women friends into ridiculous baby doll clothes, outlandish makeup, and hairstyles that seemed to live lives of their own on the tops of their heads. Something once written about another legendary beauty, Marlene Dietrich, popped into my mind: "She will never be old, because she was never young."

The face was familiar, but familiar in the same way that enabled one to recognize a piece of Hellenic sculpture. As in all of the likenesses that have come down from antiquity, there was something vaguely androgynous about this beautiful head. It could have served equally well as a model for Apollo as for Aphrodite. However, the body was distinctly female. She was wearing a flowing pale blue tie-dyed caftan, but there was no confusion about the fluid, feminine curves beneath it.

Despite the first name, none of us recognized Mrs. Kaplan as the renowned brunette Carmen who had been one of the most successful and highly paid models of the Forties, Fifties, and early Sixties. Tall and of incredibly regal carriage, she seemed to float through the group. She said very little, but her effect was unlike that of many other mute beauties: One did not grow accustomed to her looks and go about one's own business, ignoring them. There was a compulsive glancing back. She had an ineffable extra dimension, a presence, that thing so often defined as "star quality." Even in silent repose, it was felt by everybody in the room. The evening was made memorable by it and so stood out from the parties ad nauseam that are a part of the Hamptons scene.

Only later did we learn that Carmen's silence was not caused by shyness or a lack of anything to say. Although this ravishing creature would superficially seem able to command what she wished of life, she was traumatized, going through a devastating divorce and plagued by enormous doubts about herself, her looks, her future. She did not know who she was, or where she was in her life. At forty-two, she felt old, and used up, and purposeless.

Carmen spent many weekends with her friends the Leytesses, and we got to know her. Through the succeeding summers, we could see the change in her. It was nothing rapid, a slow and doubtlessly painful process, like a butterfly gradually emerging from the chrysalis. Far from the distant and silent beauty she at first had seemed, Carmen was warm, tough, responsive, opinionated, and possessed a near-Rabelaisian sense of humor.

During these seasons, I saw two things she did automatically and without flourish or ostentation: keeping in shape and helping others to do the same. She swam endless laps in the pool every day. It was a joy to watch—and no wonder, for she had once been considered an Olympic potential. One of our friends had suffered a stroke, and she got him into the pool and organized a daily program of hydrotherapy. With her women friends, she was unobtrusively helpful, giving pointers and practical advice on how to look and feel their best. She organized exercise classes, redid their makeup, cut and set their hair, and even gave pedicures. Indeed, she became a one-woman spa. If anybody became discouraged and dismissed her help by saying it was easy for her, given her looks, she would reply: "Listen, it takes more

than a handful of lucky genes."

Finally, the day arrived when she said that she had to think about doing something with the rest of her life, and I suggested that she might start by writing a book. She laughed. "About what?"

"About what you've been doing every summer with all these women."

She dismissed the idea. She was still not secure enough to believe she had anything practical to offer to anybody else. Ever helpful, she added that if I thought there was a market for such a book, she had a number of friends far better qualified than she to write it with me. There was, for example, the aging courtesan whose list of husbands and lovers sounded like a combination of Dun & Bradstreet and the Almanach de Gotha. But the market was too limited for the kind of advice she was obviously best qualified to give. There was the famous beauty whose attitude toward retaining her looks through the years sounded something like a course in guerrilla warfare. There was Barbie doll at the midcentury mark who threw everything out each season and started fresh with a new set of ten commandments of "in." Finally, there was Miss Narcissa, whose idea of communication was looking at herself in a mirror as she spoke *at* you.

They were all rejected. As far as I was concerned, if there was to be such a book, it had to be by Carmen. She had made a career in fashion since she was fourteen, but she had never mistaken that career for a religious vocation. Her attitude toward self-help was practical, down-to-earth, and did not come off as an ego trip. But Carmen was not ready, and the book was deferred.

One day, we were sitting around, and Carmen said, "Modeling is the only thing I really know and like. Do you think I'd be absolutely crazy to try it again at my age?"

Crazy! It was the sanest thing I'd ever heard. I told her she was going to start a revolution:

Carmen against the cadres of the youth movement—a battle in which I knew she would prevail. For some reason, all of this enthusiasm was more frightening than encouraging, and she murmured: "I was thinking of something more along the lines of doing a little catalog work."

Her reticence seemed incredible. If anything, she was more beautiful and in better shape than ever. She also had the authority and air of wisdom that only comes with age. In an advertisement or television commercial, she would certainly be more convincing about the values of a product than any sixteen-year-old who looked as if she was playing "dress up" in her mother's clothes. But that was strictly my opinion, which admittedly was already prejudiced in favor of Carmen. I was soon to learn what I considered her modesty about her chances was but another example of the pragmatism with which she viewed the beauty business she knew so well.

Shortly after Carmen made her decision to go back to work, I was asked to be one of the judges in the Miss U.S.A. contest. Eileen Ford, the great model's agent, was also a judge that year. One day, I casually mentioned that Carmen was about to resume her career, assuming Eileen would agree it was a wonderful idea—and might even offer to handle her again. The response was quite contrary: she felt Carmen was wasting her time since she did not look old enough for the matron thing and was too old for anything else. There was no market for her. Perhaps, it was just the atmosphere of the place;

we were judging a contest in which twenty-five was considered over the hill.

Carmen's renaissance as a model did not happen overnight. At first, the only people who believed in her potential were the photographers with whom she had worked in the past. They knew her professionalism was undiminished and that what they saw in their lenses was as good if not better than ever. It took almost a year before they found clients to agree with them. But eventually, attitudes did change, and the bookings came her way.

As Carmen's career expanded, the model agencies, including Mrs. Ford's, started to send out calls for older clients. Kaylan Pickford, Rosy, and Lillian Marcuson, among others, followed in Carmen's wake. The magazines and advertising agencies had begun to realize that there was a whole world of mature women out there who did not want to join the Pepsi generation.

In August 1982, the *Ladies' Home Journal* did a cover story on the "million-dollar models." Its subjects were Carmen, Cheryl Tiegs, Christie Brinkley, and Christina Ferrare. When she read it, Carmen was slightly startled to realize that she was old enough to have been the mother of all of the other women featured in the piece. The counterrevolution was truly launched. It was suddenly becoming fashionable to act your age and to look like a healthy, beautiful example of it. Carmen finally decided she might indeed have something to write about.

ALFRED ALLAN LEWIS

INTRODUCTION

WHEN WE STARTED TO work on this book, my first thoughts were that I was not interested in writing a book about looking younger, nor was I interested in writing a book about feeling younger: I wanted to do a book about looking and feeling *better.*

Don't get me wrong—I'm not among those who say they have earned every wrinkle they have and are proud of them. That's foolish, tantamount to saying one is proud of every mistake that one has made. Nevertheless, I do think that one of the greatest errors a woman can make is to follow in the footsteps of Ponce de León and go searching for a mythical fountain of youth. Remember the tragic end to that quest: Poor Ponce was ambushed in a Florida swamp, looking not one year younger than he had been when he first started out.

I don't believe youth is wasted on the young. As far as I'm concerned, they're welcome to it. Those who have passed it and go on longing for

it seem to have forgotten what it really was like. I wouldn't go through all of that pain, ignorance, embarrassment, and discomfort again for a lifetime pass to the Bonaventure spa. I can't waste my time wishing I had it all to do over again. I would probably make the same mistakes unless I also had the wisdom, experience, and sense of the ridiculous that it's taken all of the years of my life to acquire.

Why should any of us want to relinquish the wonderful gifts that a little age has bestowed upon us in favor of being sentimental, sloppy, sappy sixteen again? No, no. I must echo Alan Jay Lerner, who, despite seven or eight wives, once had the good sense to say, "I'm glad I'm not young anymore."

Now, being better is a whole other story. I hope I'm getting better all the time, and it is only the passage of time that gives me the space in which to do it. At any rate, I'm still in there, making the effort with all of my strength. The real purpose of this book is to share with all of you the attitudes and practical steps that are part of this effort. For my younger readers, let me say it is never too early to start; and for all of my older ones, let me state unequivocally that it is never too late to start. Time is not a thief that robs you of your natural endowments. It is a gift enabling you to enhance them.

Years ago, *Harper's Bazaar* sent me on a location trip to France for a layout on the Paris couture collection (one of the great perks for a model is the amount of traveling you get to do). I met a famous vintner and asked him the secret of his world-renowned wine. His reply has become my personal credo.

"Excellence comes with time. In the grape, ripening does not mean decaying. With the finished product, maturing does not mean going bad, nor does mellowing mean stagnation. For it all to come together takes a knowing hand, work, and patience."

It has often been said that beauty begins with the skin. Metaphorically speaking, true beauty is very much like the skin, which, as we learned in school, is composed of two layers: the dermis and the epidermis. The outer layer (epidermis) is what the world sees when it looks at us. There are many cosmetic ways to improve the appearance of it, and in the course of this book I'm going to tell you all I know about that—the sum total of forty years' experience in making a career of my looks. But anything you can do with the help of makeup or surgery is only temporary—it will fade just as our lipsticks erode within a few hours. Nothing will ameliorate the epidermis with any degree of permanence unless we also deal with what is beneath it (the dermis).

What a fascinating labyrinth of nerve endings, follicles, blood, and feelings exists beneath the face with which we face the world. Nerves and feelings—intellect, instinct, emotion—these are the things with which we live far more intimately than with the faces in our mirrors. They

have much more to do with how we look to other people than do well-proportioned bodies and symmetrical features. That lavishly praised perfect oval of a head can be a bore if it's as empty as an Easter egg.

Everything is linked in the circle of feeling and looking better. We cannot look our best unless we feel good about ourselves, and we cannot feel good about ourselves unless we look our best. The marriage of the outer and inner self is the only union that cannot be put asunder.

Later, we will discuss plastic surgery. I'm all for it when there is an emotional or physical or professional need for it, but there is a catch. Whenever friends ask my advice about cosmetic surgery, I always tell them to bear one thing in mind: Your face may be lifted sky-high, but you're the same person underneath. Any change in the way others perceive you is fleeting unless the spirit of the inner woman is also lifted.

Lasting change starts inside and works its way to the surface and not the reverse. Without a positive attitude about yourself, there is no cosmetic, calisthenic, or nutritional suggestion that I or anybody else can make that will work longer than it takes to read about it. If all of the beauty, glamour, diet, and exercise books that have been sold to women had really worked, we would all be such paragons of glowing health and good looks as the world has never before beheld. That we are not these wondrous creatures means that we have been treating the often valuable information that these books may contain as if it were a Band-Aid, applying it to the surface in the hope that the "boo-boo" will go away. It is much easier to change the color of one's eye shadow than to change the tone of one's perception of oneself. Everything that I am about to share with you is true and will be of lasting help, but only if you use it to work *toward* the surface and not *on* the surface.

Diets do not work unless one permanently changes one's eating habits. At our age, a nutritionist must be consulted. Our health must last much longer than our waistlines.

Exercises do not work if they do not become a part of your daily life. Being a weekend jogger, tennis player, bicyclist, or swimmer is not enough. Indeed, these sudden spurts of physical exertion may actually be dangerous.

Makeup lessons work only on the woman who has already decided that she likes who she is and wants to improve rather than distort her own special self. The rule is, To thine own face be true.

Your face is not a canvas on which to paint Brooke Shields's features, or mine, or those of anybody else you might admire. It is a wonderful individual thing that is all your own. There is not a woman in the world who does not have at least one good feature: hair, eyes, skin, nose, lips, bone structure. Like wise investors in promising futures, let's make the most of our assets while diminishing our liabilities at the same time.

We all have defects, which the wrong cosmetics only accentuate (*wrong* can generally be interpreted as too much). Without the right makeup, I have a peculiarly Picassoesque look: One eye is slightly higher than the other, and my lips are too thin. That's why I hoot at the "legendary beauty" appellation; it seems to me that "cubist painting" would be a more accurate description. But do you know what I do to correct these defects? Nothing. The worst thing would be to paint on a mouth where there is none. As for my eyes, I actually accentuate them. They're my best feature. It would be all wrong to try to correct what nature has decreed is uncorrectable.

I think it was Dr. Samuel Johnson who said that by the time we're fifty, we get the faces we deserve—meaning that all of our vices and virtues are reflected in them. I do agree that we get what we deserve, but I don't think it has anything to do with our ethics. Some of the wickedest people I know look perfectly marvelous and, alas, some of the nicest look terrible.

There are no scarlet letters. The face is not a mirror of morality. It merely reflects self-esteem. If you hold yourself in high regard, no matter how unacceptable your behavior, you will take care of yourself, and the shining countenance will be the face you've earned. Apathy and laziness will likewise be rewarded with the dull and lackluster appearance that they merit.

I am going to tell you a little bit about my life, for it is my credential, and the experiences in it are the only things that equip me to tell you anything that might be of benefit in yours. It has not been without its share of excitement and variety. I've been a wife too often and a mother not often enough, and a career person, and a homemaker. I've had my allowance of disasters as well as triumphs.

When I was very young and just embarking on my career, I felt fortunate that I photographed well, but I was bewildered when people did not react positively to the child I still was. My conviction that all of life was a matter of luck led naturally to insecurity. Each day began with fear. What if this was the day the luck ran out? Where would I be? Who would want me? And inevitably the day did arrive when all of my fears seemed to become reality. My luck had run out, and I felt utterly lost. My career was finished, my child was ill, and the man I wanted most in the world no longer wanted me. The years of living on my face and figure had imposed a regimen that kept me looking good, but I thought it was a hollow shell that would disintegrate with time, for there was nothing left inside to sustain it. At forty-three I felt old and burnt-out.

I had lived too long being other people's fantasy, trying to please them, trying to live up to their image of me. Call it a midlife crisis, call it what you will, but it was a time for reassessment. I hesitantly embarked upon a rite of passage far more painful than the sexual one of my adolescence. The first thing that became apparent was that I must forget the fear of being thought vain and become the most important person in my life. Only by beginning to think well of myself would I have the courage to reshape my life, to become important to other people again, to enter new relationships as an equal partner.

After you have done all of the things necessary to establish a career, after the children are grown, after the love affairs and marriages have been defined as enduring or over, only one thing remains, and that is the thread that bound all of the rest together. Yourself. You have earned the right to your indulgences. You can give yourself permission to become the most important person in your life.

The first step is to place a high value on you. You've spent a lifetime giving love to others, pampering them, and following rules you never made to attain goals you never set. Now, at the height of your feminine powers, at the age of renaissance, you must begin to love and pamper yourself. The one rule that remains is self-actualization. I've been fortunate because the art of pampering, polishing, buffing my physical self has been one of the tools of my trade. I have taken it for granted, but it should become a part of every woman's life. I had to develop an individual look, or there would be no reason to hire me instead of any of dozens of other equally professional and photogenic models.

I want to share all of the things I have learned in these forty years of preparing myself for the cameras. My goal is to help you to find a style of your own that will free you from the slavery of following the fashions of others. Along the way, I hope you will discover, as I have, that all the old adages that seemed so trite when we were young are really true. Today really *is* the most important day in your life. There *is* power in positive thinking. Every day in every way, you *can* become better and better.

STAYING BEAUTIFUL

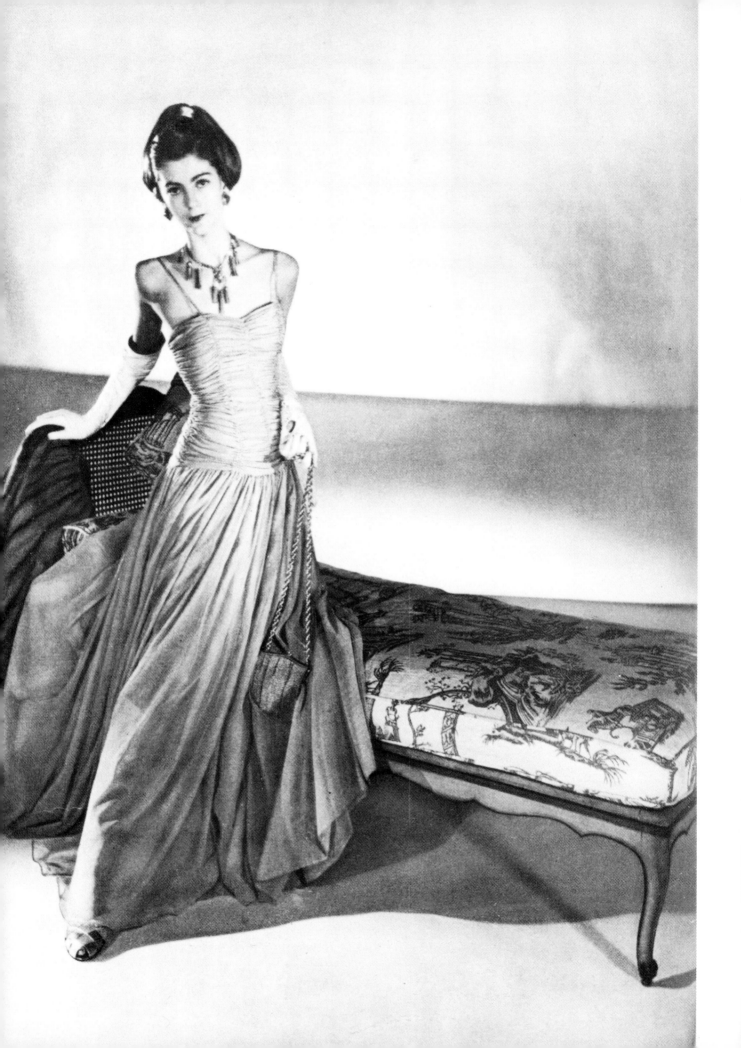

1

MY LIFE

WHEN I WAS YOUNGER, I used to hate it when people said that Carmen's life was a real Cinderella story. Now, with age and a little objectivity, I can see what they meant. I must admit, with all due and undue respect to the men in my life, there has been nothing that could remotely pass for a Prince Charming (some toads and some charmers, but no princes). And I've sat out more than a few dances. But it has been a ball.

My mother, Margaret (called Peggy), was a Hungarian dancer. She was pastry pretty but so practical that as a child I often suspected the cook had left out most of the sugar. Papa, Joseph Dell'Orefice, was an Italian violinist of the traditional tall-dark-and-handsome variety. He

The Horst picture for which he wrote some very flattering words. *(Horst)*

provided all the sweet sounds in my young life, a kind of ubiquitous Muzak that underscored my daydreams.

Mama immigrated to this country when she was in her early adolescence and landed in Detroit, where she had some family. It was later determined she had a genius-level IQ, and she taught herself English by starting with *A* and working through *zymurgy* in Webster's dictionary. It was not long before she was winning citywide spelling bees. Need I add that, in addition to being extremely bright, she was a very determined young lady?

When mama was sixteen, she won a dance scholarship and came to New York City to study with Albertina Rasch. She eventually got a job as one of the Roxyettes, the forerunners of the Rockettes. The Roxyettes danced in the lavish stage productions that alternated with the films at the almost inconceivably baroque

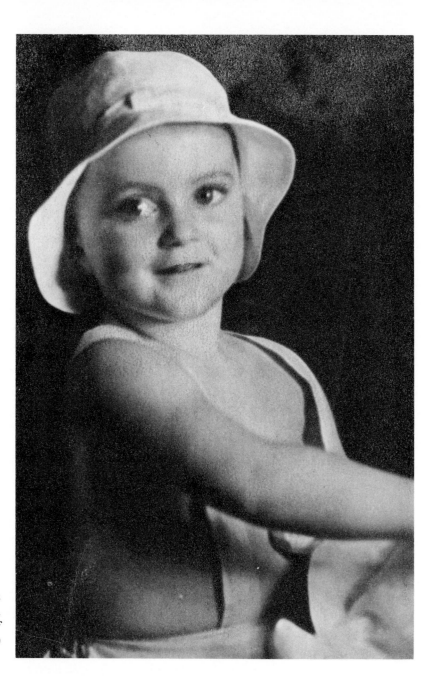

Me at age 3. If you don't count pregnancy, the last time I was a stylish stout. (*Collection of Carmen*)

Roxy Theater. Until its demolition, it was one of the city's more imposing landmarks, standing at the corner of West Fiftieth Street and Seventh Avenue.

My father was first violinist in the great concert orchestra at the same theater. He was part of a distinguished musical family. His cousin, Eugenio, was choirmaster for the Metropolitan Opera, and his brother, my uncle Enzo, had been Enrico Caruso's coach and accompanist at the time of his New York debut. My grandfa-

ther had been the head of the Naples Conservatory of Music, as had been his father before him, who was also the composer of several popular operas of the period.

Descended from this classical musical lineage, it was only natural that papa was more than a little disdainful of what he was playing in the Roxy pit. The boredom caused his attention to wander up to the productions on the stage above him. Being Italian and considering himself a born connoisseur of such things, he singled out and became enamored of the best pair of legs on that stage long before confronting their owner, my mother, face-to-face. The face that faced his was not bad either, and they began to "keep company," as it was euphemistically put in those days. The closeness of that company led to marriage and a radical alteration in the figure carried by those legs papa loved so well. She was pregnant, and they both lost their jobs. I was born soon after, on June 3, 1931, on Welfare Island. The name of that not very romantic isle tells the whole story. Mama was twenty-one and papa nearly twenty years older. It was during the depression, and they were broke.

It is said that the first five years of a child's life determine the shape of the rest of that life. Certainly whatever toughness, resilience, and endurance I have were formed during those years. So was the ability to fantasize and to shield and protect those fantasies with every ounce of my fragile strength. Nobody could ever take away my dreams; nobody could ever spoil them. In fact, my constant fantasizing might have turned me into a first-class psychotic had it not been for the good fortune of looks that became a discipline, and a way of life, and a career even before I reached puberty.

It may sound melodramatic, but the beauty that other people saw in me (while I still disbelieved it) may well have saved my sanity. Perhaps that is why I have always appreciated this accident of genes, or gift of God, or whatever it is, and carefully attempted to preserve it, using all of the knowledge and tricks I've gathered through the years in which it has been the source of my fame and my fortune and, yes, my salvation. It has not been through any sense of personal vanity that I have done this (although I have that, or I would never have attempted this book); it is because beauty was the life preserver thrown to me when I most needed it, and I have no intention of throwing it away, not while I'm still in the swim of things.

And so, I was born into the worst depression the world has ever known, to parents whose relationship paralleled the economy. It was grim. They would meet and live together on and off, mostly off, in the hope of some sort of recovery, which proved as unsettling as the stock market of the period. Papa took whatever jobs he could find—generally with second-rate touring orchestras—and sent home what money he could spare, which was not much.

Mama put aside any dreams she might have had of becoming a great dancer and took the only work for which she was qualified, as a housekeeper or waitress. I was either boarded with relatives not much better off than we were, or at foster homes, or tucked away in the attics of homes where she was working as a housekeeper or nursemaid. There was always an unspoken agreement between mama and me: I was not to appear to be livelier or brighter or prettier than the children of the home we were living in, or they would throw us out into the streets. After a while I stopped thinking it was possible for me to be any of those things, and that was how we managed to survive.

Then, when I was six, everything seemed to change. Can anybody believe that six can be a golden age? For me, it was a year I still recall as one of the brightest and best in a lifetime that has spanned almost half a century longer. Papa had come back to us, bringing with him his gifts of sunshine, and love, and music, and laughter. We were still very poor, living in what was little better than a slum in the Jackson Heights section of Queens. It couldn't have mattered less to me. I was so happy, and what happy child with a penny in her pocket for candy knows anything about economics?

It was during that year that I began to go to school, which I adored, and it was during the summer of that year that I experienced my first taste of public admiration. I must admit I also adored that.

Mama was a native of a landlocked country, but with perverse determination she turned herself into an excellent swimmer. She must have taught me how to swim while I was still an infant, for I cannot remember a time when I could not swim. During my wonderful sixth summer, we lived very close to the Astoria Swimming Pool. It was actually an amphitheater with an outdoor Olympic-size pool. Vic Zobel staged water shows there that were quite famous at the time. One day, he saw me dive and swim and obtained my parents' permission to use me in that year's production.

There was a moment in the show when a spotlight beamed on a little girl standing on a platform some sixteen feet above the water. Her back was arched, her hands stretched stiffly above her head. As she raised herself on tiptoe, the audience became silent and strained forward, astonished that this frail, skinny little thing was actually going to dive from that height. I knew I had them and tried never to let them down. The dive was as perfect and graceful as I could possibly make it. As my head emerged from the water, the thrilling applause penetrated the rubber swimming cap to every part of me, and I felt a sense of accomplishment and love I had never experienced before and have seldom equaled since.

The show was my shining hour until an accident occurred. One day, I misjudged the dive, and as my head hit the water, I heard, more than felt, something crack. I had broken my nose. It was very painful, but they packed it and the bleeding stopped. There was no thought of surgery; we couldn't afford it. The bone mended on its own, and that was the end of it except for some sporadic bouts of difficult breathing during bad weather.

Inevitably, my temperamental parents separated again, and mama and I were on our own. In my child's mind, it seemed we always lived alongside places and never in them, as we moved from Wood*side,* to Sunny*side,* to Bay*side.* We went wherever my mother could get a rent-free apartment in exchange for doing janitor's chores. Before leaving for her regular job, she would sweep out the halls and light the fires for the coal furnaces. In a way, it was the start of my alleged fairy-tale existence. I had a very early acquaintanceship with the cinders part of Cinderella.

I can remember all of my own young dreams, but only recently have I realized that my mother had not forsaken *her* dreams; she had simply transferred them and intended to live out her dream of the dance through me. That was why she used papa's connections in the music world to get me an audition for a scholarship at the school of Vjaschaslav and Maria Swoboda. The Swobodas had the best ballet school of the period and prepared all of the young dancers for the Ballet Russe de Monte Carlo.

On that first day, I executed a *plié* naturally, without awkward knees or elbows. The Swobodas agreed to give me the scholarship if I would promise to come to class every day. That was no chore. I was mad about dancing and could hardly wait for Saturdays, when I could take two or three classes. I was a wraith with energy to spare—for which mama's cooking could be thanked. She was a health-food devotee long before it became a fad. The mainstays of our diet were whole grains, fruits, and vegetables prepared simply and *al dente.*

In the ballet classes, I was, if not a swan, at least a cygnet. In public school, I was an off-horse—too tall, too skinny, with crooked teeth (more about them later) and straight hair in an era when masses of curls were all the rage. If I think about it, I guess I never was in fashion except as a business. Don't get me wrong—when I look at those old photographs, I realize that I was a pretty child by any adult standards. Still, I was ugly by other children's standards, and that was what counted. I longed to be short and dainty and look like Shirley Temple. That was the definition of *pretty* back then. Ruffles

At age 10. Too tall, too thin, and already looking too old for my contemporaries. (*Collection of Carmen*)

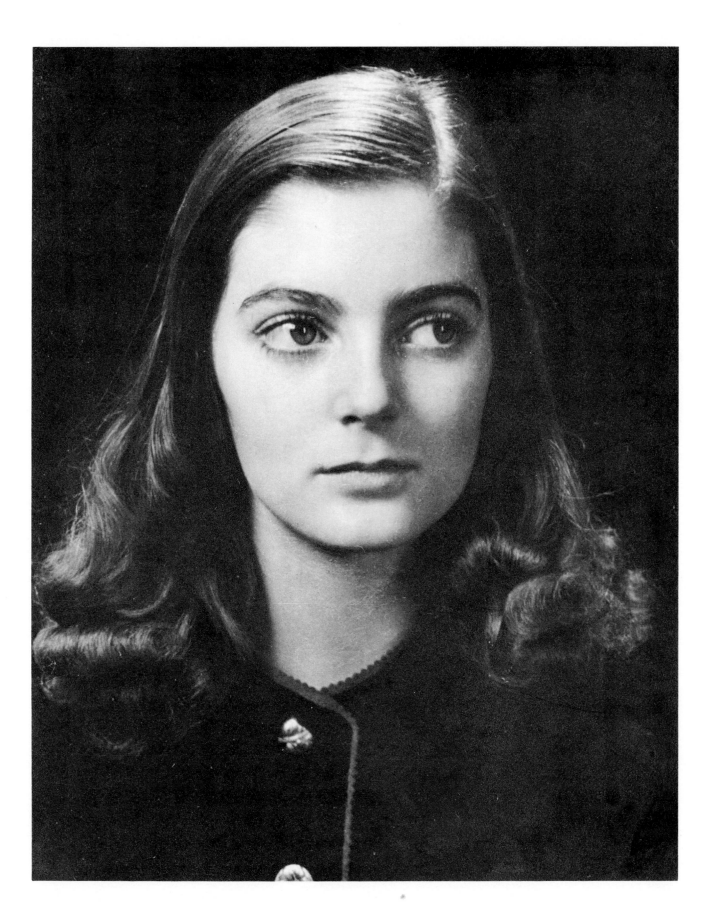

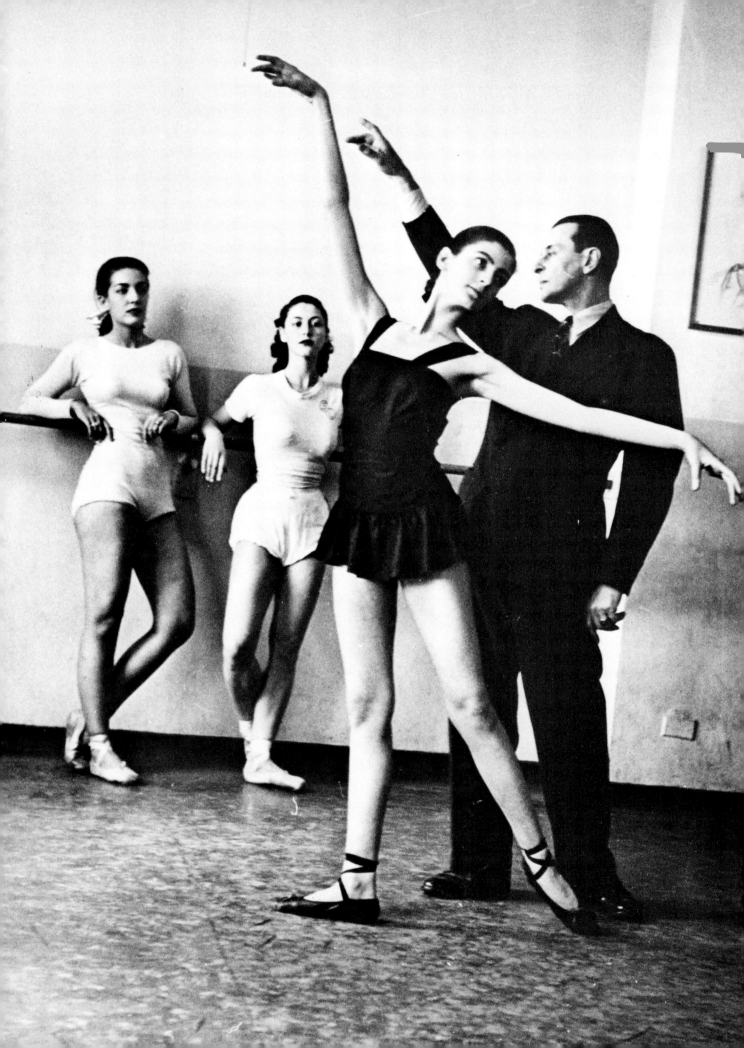

and bows rather than the jeans and sweaters of today. It occurs to me that a kid who looks like Shirley Temple in 1985 must feel every bit as out of it as I did not looking like her in 1939.

Mama was a wonderful seamstress and stayed up long into the night making me little dresses that were all pleats and flairs and sashes and lace insets. They only accentuated my long legs and made me look still more awkward to my classmates. I might have been sensational in a button-down shirt with tails flapping over blue denim, but movie dreams and school authorities conspired to decree that this was not the way a girl child was supposed to look. At the time, I agreed with them; like all children, I longed to conform, to look like a magazine illustration. Only long after I became a magazine illustration did I discover how distorting popular fashion could be to my body and personal style.

When I was eleven years old, mama and I finally moved into Manhattan. We found a small apartment at 900 Third Avenue. It was on the fourth floor, and although the Third Avenue elevated line rattled by day and night, no elevator went up and down in our building. It did not matter. That fourth-floor walk-up was heaven to me. It meant I did not have to waste time taking the subways into the city for my ballet classes and could take two classes on weekdays and three on Saturdays. The Swobodas thought I had great promise if only I would stop growing. Male dancers were generally of medium height at best, and a ballerina who hovered at six feet, *au point,* did not have much of a future.

Taking classes with me at that time was one little boy who would later prove a stellar exception to that rule about short males. His sister was also in the classes, and every day their formidable French mother would sit at the back of

the room with knitting needles clicking away rather like Mme. De Farge. I think she enrolled the boy only to save money on a baby-sitter for him while she took her daughter to class. He was a funny-looking kid with a wide gap between his front teeth, a turned-up nose, and a cowlick that always stood straight up, but he was having a wonderful time jumping around, and when he grew up, Jacques d'Amboise became a pretty formidable dancer—and divinely tall.

The next year, I was stricken with rheumatic fever and ordered to remain in bed. The worst part of that confinement was that with muscles totally relaxed, I seemed to grow faster than ever—three inches in less than a year. My mother managed to nurse me, run the house, and hold on to a couple of jobs, but after nine months she thought enough was more than enough. Although the physicians of the period said "No exercise, no movement," she got me out of bed and bundled me off on the Fifty-seventh Street crosstown bus to Seventh Avenue and the old Park Central Hotel, which had an Olympic swimming pool.

On wobbly legs, I looked more like a Giacometti than a potential Giselle, but as I've said, I cannot remember a time when I was not able to swim, and despite the illness, I must still have had pretty good form. The woman in charge of the pool, Ethelda Bleibtry, was a former Olympic champion and constantly on the lookout for future candidates for the team. She saw potential in me and told my mother she would coach me, but only if I was permitted to come to train with her every day. All thoughts of medical warnings flew right out of mama's head. It was like a scholarship, and she was never one to turn down giveaways for her daughter. From total confinement to bed, I moved overnight to daily swimming lessons, and my strength rapidly returned. What is amazing is that what my mother did against all medical advice back then is exactly what is often prescribed now for similar ailments.

In ballet class with Vjaschaslav Swoboda. *(Leonard McCombe)*

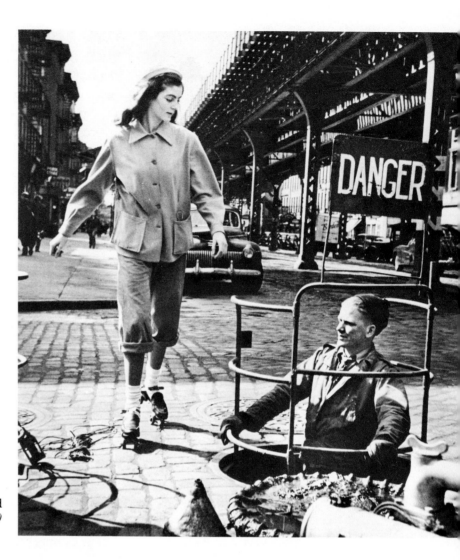

The demon roller skater of Third Avenue. *(Leonard McCombe)*

I loved to roller-skate, and once liberated from bed, my feet were in my skates almost before they were in my bobby socks. In the heart of heavy midtown Manhattan traffic, this tall, skinny apparition on wheels, usually pulled along by Honey, my lively cocker spaniel, must have been a sight eccentric enough to make Boy George look like a preppie. I couldn't have cared less. Those eight wheels were my freedom. I still love it. Recently, my favorite photographer, Norman Parkinson, took a picture of me skating across Westminster Bridge in London, dressed in a gorgeous ball gown designed by the Emanuels, Princess Diana's favorite dressmakers.

When I wasn't on skates, the Fifty-seventh Street crosstown bus was my personal chariot. From Third Avenue, where we lived, it carried me to all of the meaningful places in my young life: to the Swoboda studio, the Park Central swimming pool, and later to the Lodge Professional Children's School. It was on this bus that I was supposedly "discovered." In the many publicity accounts through the years, it's been called the fashion model's equivalent of Lana Turner at the soda fountain, and it was no more the truth of how I got started than it was of Lana's start. What follows is what actually happened.

I was on my way home from the pool one day

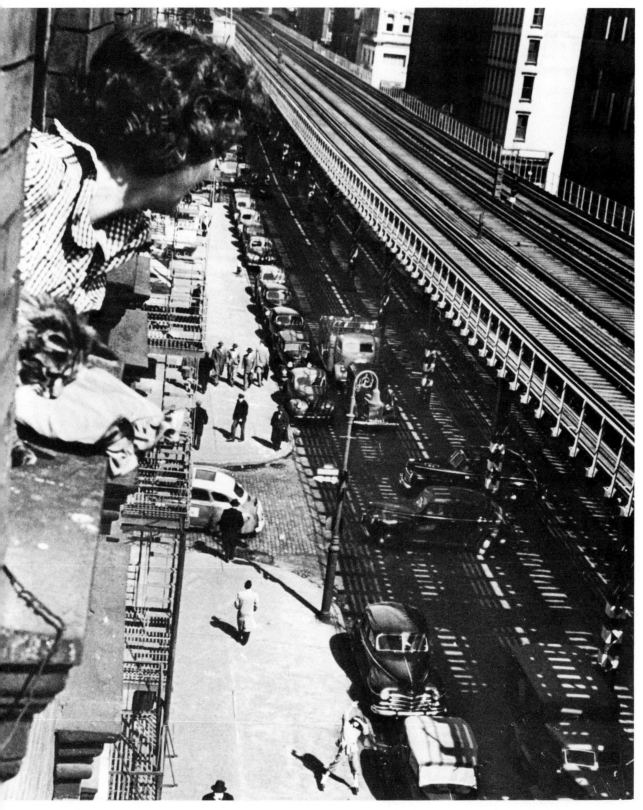

Mama calling me to supper from our fourth-floor walk-up. Lung power substituted for the phone we did not own. *(Leonard McCombe)*

when a woman approached me on the bus. She was the wife of a staff photographer for *Harper's Bazaar* and explained that she thought her husband might be interested in taking some test shots of me. She wanted to call my mother for permission, and when I told her we had no telephone, she suggested that my mother call her. It was another "scholarship," and mama raced down those four flights two steps at a time to get to the pay phone in the local drugstore.

The photographer took me out to Jones Beach and photographed me on my roller skates and larking about on the beach wearing the most beautiful collection of sweaters I had ever seen. I was having a wonderful time but had no thoughts of this having any relationship to a career. In my mind, the future was as crystal clear as that day at the beach: I was going to be the first prima ballerina to win a gold medal for swimming in the Olympic Games.

A short time later, mama got a very polite letter from an editor at *Bazaar*. It informed her that she had a charming and well-mannered child who was totally unphotogenic. Mama framed it and hung it in a place of honor—in our bathroom.

My godfather, Gregory D'Alessio, taught at the Art Students League and was a prominent cartoonist. His series, "These Women," appeared regularly in *The New Yorker*. When mama told Gregory about the letter, he studied me and said with a twinkle in his eyes, "Well—you know—I don't think she's so ugly."

I'll never forget his words because it seemed to me I really was ugly. Other girls my age were beginning to have figures, and all I had was a rib cage. My chest was so flat, it was concave. I had the broad shoulders of a swimmer and the erect carriage of a dancer, but I had no hips and a backside that was more like pita bread than buns. But if Gregory thought I wasn't so ugly, it could be true—perhaps I wasn't. He didn't say I was pretty, but I hadn't expected that. Being not so ugly was enough to make my day.

Gregory played in a classical guitar group.

One of the other musicians was married to Carol Philips, who worked for *Vogue*. Gregory's wife and my godmother, Hilda Terry (also a well-known cartoonist), suggested that he ask Carol to have a look at me. Another test I'll probably fail, I thought, but I was willing to walk to hell and back if there was the remotest chance of approval. Two weeks later, I was summoned to the offices of Condé Nast, publishers of *Vogue, Glamour,* and several other glossy and successful "women's" magazines. They had to dispatch a secretary to fetch me, because, of course, we had no phone. It was not only a matter of poverty; it was the times—World War II had just ended and there was a shortage of telephones.

The offices of *Vogue* were indescribably sleek, and filled with smart young women whose heads in those days were encased, indoors and out, in what were described as "cunning little hats." They spoke with such debutante drawls that were their cheeks not so hollow, one would have sworn their mouths were filled with marbles. Their conversations were punctuated by a series of adjectives—*fabulous,* and *fantastic,* and *absurd*—designated as "in" by those doyennes of fashion, Diana Vreeland and Carmel Snow. Their English was seasoned with French phrases in the style of those who are insecure in both languages.

I think I may safely say that mine was a singular entrance into that sanctum sanctorum of chic. My hair was in pigtails and my feet in bobby socks and brown-and-white oxfords. Although I wasn't wearing my skates, I had insisted on bringing Honey because I was afraid I'd need a friend. As the secretary towed me along, I tugged at Honey's leash, desperately praying she would not have an accident of the sort I was certain never occurred in those enameled corridors.

Carol Philips was a warm and beautiful blonde, so beautiful I wondered what chance I had if somebody who looked like her was sitting behind a desk instead of posing in front of

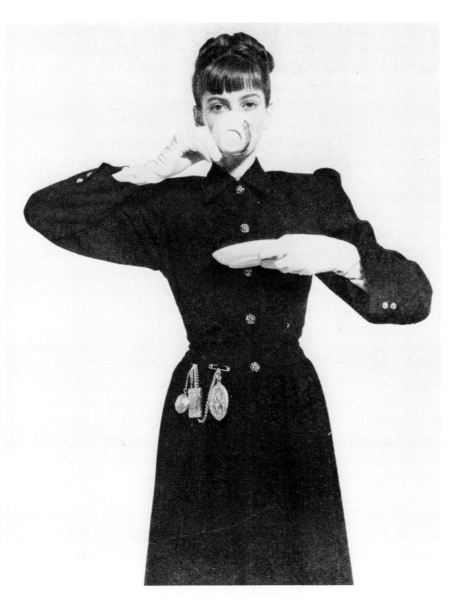

The first *Vogue* photograph that convinced mama that there was something terribly wrong with my face. *(Clifford Coffin)*

a camera. Today, Carol is the president of Clinique and still warm, and beautiful, and blonde.

She tilted my face this way and that and studied the bony length of me. I was too frightened to speak, but Carol must have liked what she saw, because before I knew it, I was in the *Vogue* studios, clad in beautiful clothes, my face painted by an editor (there were no makeup artists in those days), and sitting for a photographer named Clifford Coffin, who was mad, and wonderful, and brutally objective. He told me he did not like my mouth—it was too thin—but

that I did have beautiful eyes. He solved the problem by posing me with a raised cup of tea that obscured every feature except the eyes and ears, which he said were too large, but which he could do nothing about. The picture bore him out, and it came as no surprise, for my mother had already told me my ears were like sedan chairs.

Coffin really socked it to me about my pluses and minuses. I was too frightened to hear any of the good things he said; it seemed that only what was wrong with me was again being underlined. I was fourteen and unnoticed by my peers—which is to say, the boys never noticed me. Believe me, I would gladly have traded oceans of Condé Nast approval for one smile from the corner grocer's gorgeous son.

There were seven pages scattered through two issues of the magazine from that first sitting. When they appeared, however, all my mother seemed able to see was that cup and saucer. There had to be something terribly wrong with my face if the photographer wanted to cover it. She decided it was my teeth and marched me off to a dentist to have braces put on them—which, if you think about it, is a very odd thing to do to a girl embarking on a modeling career. For the next four years, I never smiled in a picture. It gave rise to an early image of remote and glamorous mystery that set me apart from the other teen models. The truth was, I had a mouthful of hardware, and nobody wanted me to open it.

Carol Philips later said that when she saw those first photographs, she was very upset. She knew she had discovered a star, but wondered if she wanted to take responsibility for pushing anybody so young and inexperienced into the cynical world of high fashion. That was long before the era of the Pill and Brooke Shields; a fourteen-year-old girl was still considered an innocent child. In my case, it was the truth—I hadn't even started to menstruate. But Gregory had told Carol how much we needed the money, and she felt she could not deny me the opportunity. I was offered $7.50 an hour, which is what some models make a minute these days, but it seemed like a fortune to mama and me.

Actually, then as now, the big money was in commercial modeling, and the exclusive contract we signed with Condé Nast did not permit me to do any outside work. In that period, the Condé Nast "girls" were a breed apart, acolytes in the temple of high fashion. The publishers did not want us to sully our faces in the hundreds of advertising pages that were the actual source of the magazine's profits. In publications such as *Vogue*, the ratio was usually four advertising pages to one page of editorial. We had to be the special, distant goddesses reserved for those few precious pages that were not for sale. It did not matter that away from the cameras, we chewed gum, had cramps, had disastrous marriages and love affairs, did not know how to handle the money we earned during our few fleeting years as stars, and seldom got as far as a high-school diploma. In front of the cameras, we had to look as if we had never heard of a toilet, much less used one. God, and the editors who were his representatives on earth, forbid that we be seen endorsing a deodorant or lingerie. All this was during a time when those same editors were rushing out to install bidets in New York apartments, presumably as conversation pieces.

Within my first few months in the *Vogue* studios, I worked for most of the greatest fashion photographers of the period: Beaton, Horst, Penn, Blumenfeld, Joffe, Rawlings, and Scavullo. They all seemed to want "little Carmen," which was Penn's name for me. The strange thing was that although I was the youngest model in the house, I was never seen in the editorial pages devoted to junior fashion. From the beginning, I was dressed only in the clothes meant to appeal to women in their thirties and older.

The great photographer Francesco Scavullo described what I was like when only a few years out of grammar school and still an off-horse— but a well-paid one by then.

"The first time I photographed Carmen, in 1948, for *Seventeen*, they told me she was too old for the magazine. She was sixteen. But nothing about her look was childlike. It was high fashion, sophisticated, soignée—a woman's look. At sixteen, five feet nine inches tall, she was a *femme*

The Beaton photograph that remains one of my favorites of the early period of my career. *(Cecil Beaton)*

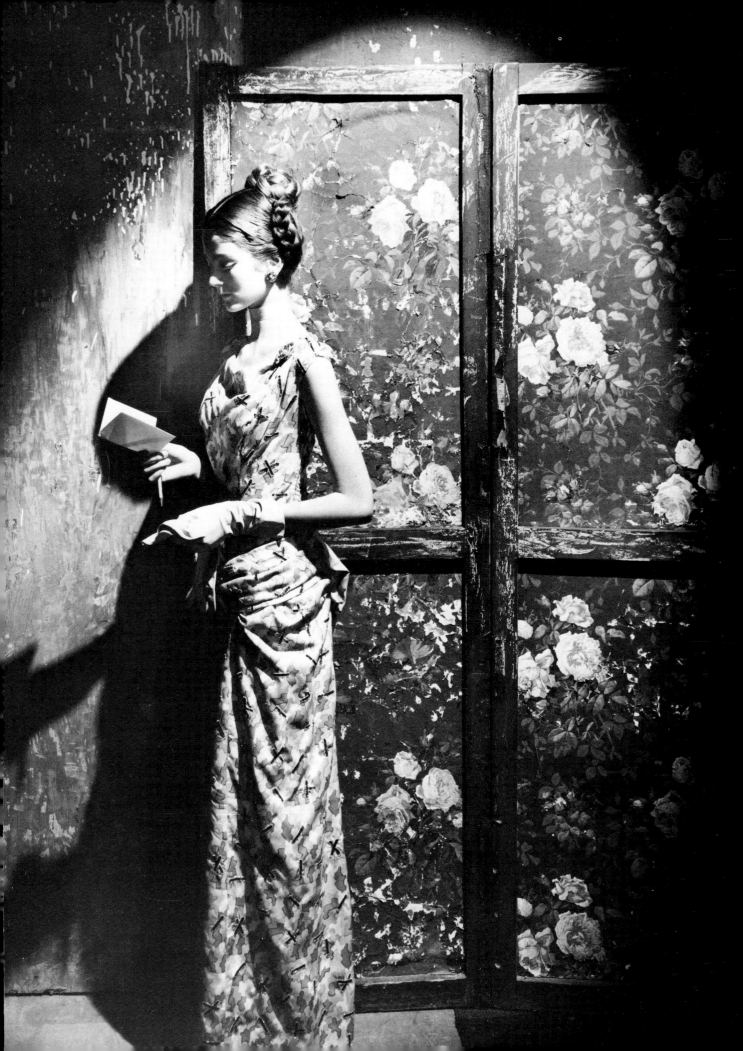

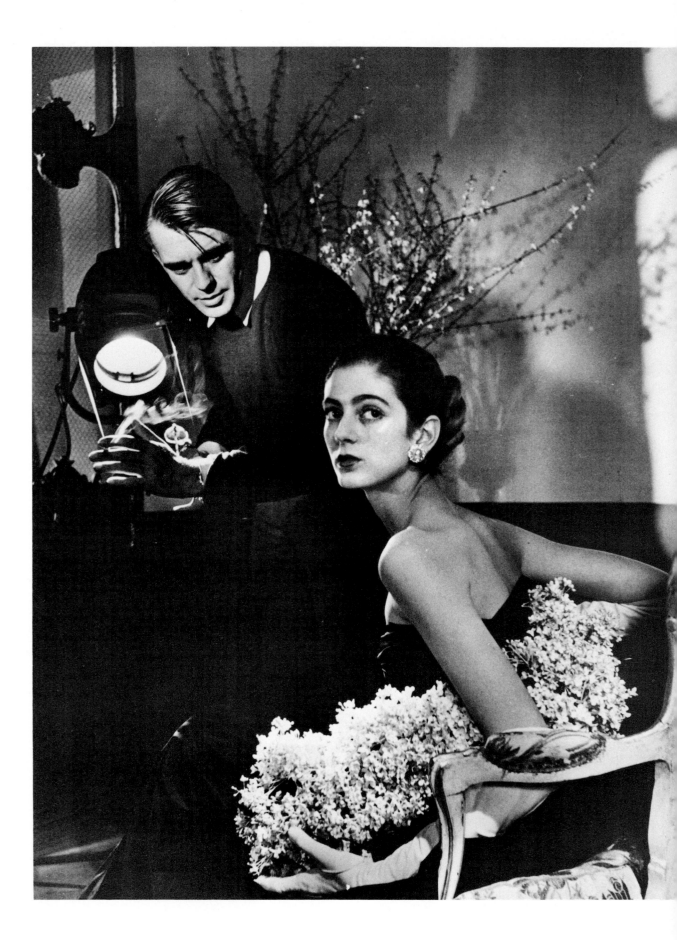

de monde who didn't even have a bosom yet.

"I tried to make her a little girl. I did Alice in Wonderland hair. I had her stand very demurely. And we got a good picture. But they were right—Carmen never did belong in *Seventeen.* But at *Vogue*! They put those Mainbocher clothes on this infant and she'd look as though she'd been born in them."

What Frank could not have realized was that at that age I would far rather have been *Seventeen* than *Vogue.* I hadn't found my own style. But today, how I wish I owned some of those Mainbochers! I'd still be wearing them, and they'd still look terrific. He was one of those rare designers who were never concerned with having their clothes in fashion, and so they were never out of it. Style was everything, and his customers knew who they were and how they looked their best. It did not matter how "new" M. Dior's look was, they remained faithful to Main. Isn't it strange how dated that "new look" has become, how much a part of the past, and how timeless Mainbocher remains? I've said it before: New is not better, it is only newer.

Cecil Beaton was the first man ever to make me feel beautiful. He took what remains my favorite photograph of all those of the early years. They simulated a garden in the studio with hundreds of pots of ferns and flowering shrubs. I sat in a wicker chair wearing a white eyelet dress designed by Sophie and carrying a matching parasol. The lighting was totally unrealistic—lots of blues and roses—but Beaton was not interested in showing off the dress. To him, the mood was the important thing, and the result has always reminded me of an impressionist painting of a young girl in a long-ago garden illuminated only by the evanescent light of a given moment on an early summer evening.

One day, Beaton asked me if I would like to

An early *Vogue* sitting with the great and gentle and very handsome Horst. *(Leonard McCombe)*

earn some extra money posing for a friend of his who was a well-known painter. The name, Salvador Dali, meant nothing to either my mother or me. The extra money meant everything. Dali wanted me nude from the waist up. As I had absolutely no sign of a bust, we agreed, rationalizing that I had nothing to hide. When the painting was finished, I was thrilled to discover that Dali had provided what nature had neglected.

Dali lived and worked in a suite at the St. Regis Hotel. The floor was littered with preliminary sketches of the animals that would appear along with my figure in the picture he was painting. I coveted those wonderful sketches, and one day he said I could have them in lieu of my modeling fee. My mother would not permit me to accept Dali's offer. In our financial condition, $7.50 an hour was worth a great deal more than a set of original Dali drawings.

Cecil Beaton also lived at the St. Regis. It was about this time, or shortly after, that he and Dali decorated widely photographed suites for the hotel, which were considered very innovative. I wonder what eventually became of them. The hotel management was probably no more prescient about these works of art than my mother had been about the Dali drawings. And while collecting the photographs for this book, I discovered that the magazines were just as neglectful about their works of art. They had hired the very finest photographers of the twentieth century. The pictures they took raised the public's consciousness of photographs as works of art. But instead of preserving them or giving them to the collections of schools and museums or even returning them to the photographers, during that period before the copyright laws were changed and they were forced to, the publishers destroyed them to make room in their archives for editorial memos on the length of a hem.

Each day, after my sessions with Dali were over, Beaton would pick me up and take me to lunch across Fifty-fifth Street at Le Pavillon, which was then the finest restaurant in the city. The food was so delicious, I knew it had to be sinful, and I relished every morsel of it even if I didn't know the names of the things I was eating. It was the beginning of a gastronomic education with Beaton as tutor. During those afternoons, I was given a crash course in so many of the small but finer arts under his tutelage.

Beaton was slim, suave, and sophisticated, and so sweet to me. On some days, he would be clad with such unutterable elegance that Savile Row would have trembled. On others, he would turn up in flowing black cape, dashing borsalino, and fulsome ties in patterns that seemed to be at war with the equally colorful patterns of his jackets and shirts—such a dashing bohemian that Savile Row would have shuddered while Chelsea sighed. All of this—the names of these faraway places, who frequented them, the philosophy of haute couture, the intricacies of gourmet cooking, what painting meant, why photography was an art—all of this, I began to learn during those languid afternoons sunk into the red plush banquettes beneath murals of a France as fanciful as the settings for a Beaton photograph.

The restaurant is still there, but now it is called La Côte Basque, and memories of that enchanted, too brief time in my life are evoked each time I dine there. Although the murals and banquettes have been refurbished, they are roughly as they were almost forty years ago, and the food is still sinfully good. Time has not jaded my taste for it, but the ever-encroaching spread of middle age has enforced a certain abstemiousness.

Horst was another photographer I remember with great fondness. He was very gentle and considerate of my feelings, never patronizing or talking down to me as to a child. His photographs were always very elegant depictions of a cool creature dressed and posed in worldly attitudes far beyond my limited experience. The clothes were held to my thin frame by rows of clothespins running down their rear, and the slightly bosomy protuberances were created by tissue paper wadded into the bodices. I looked at the finished pictures and saw no relationship to the real me. Although it would have been thrilling to be that romantic-looking girl, dressed in those gorgeous clothes, on her way to some romantic rendezvous, she was Horst's fantasy. My real assignations were at the grocery store under the Third Avenue el, where the grocer's handsome son continued to ignore the skinny kid with braces on her teeth who was constantly roller-skating by.

Models were not celebrities in those days. The public seldom knew the names attached to the familiar face of a Muriel Maxwell or a Bettina Bollagard. Recognition by name arrived only when the name was romantically linked to that of some dashing playboy—and, believe me, those boys really knew how to play and dash; they were almost never caught.

When a name was used in a photographic caption in the Forties, you could be sure it belonged to a socialite, or debutante, or actress, or celebrity, a woman so eager for the publicity and prestige that came with appearing in *Vogue* that she posed for hours without pay in clothes she did not own. It was amazing to find my first year as a *Vogue* model celebrated with the appearance of my name along with my picture.

Four of the magazine's leading photographers were asked to photograph and describe their ideal beauties. Dorian Leigh and I were the only models in the batch, and I was the only one who was actually a *Vogue* girl. Dorian was chosen by Penn. Blumenfeld selected Mrs. Cushing Mortimer, who was later to become the world's best-dressed woman as Mrs. William ("Babe") Paley. At the time, she was *Vogue*'s resident socialite/editor/beauty. Rawlings chose the

---

1946. The first Horst photograph of me to appear in *Vogue*. (Horst)

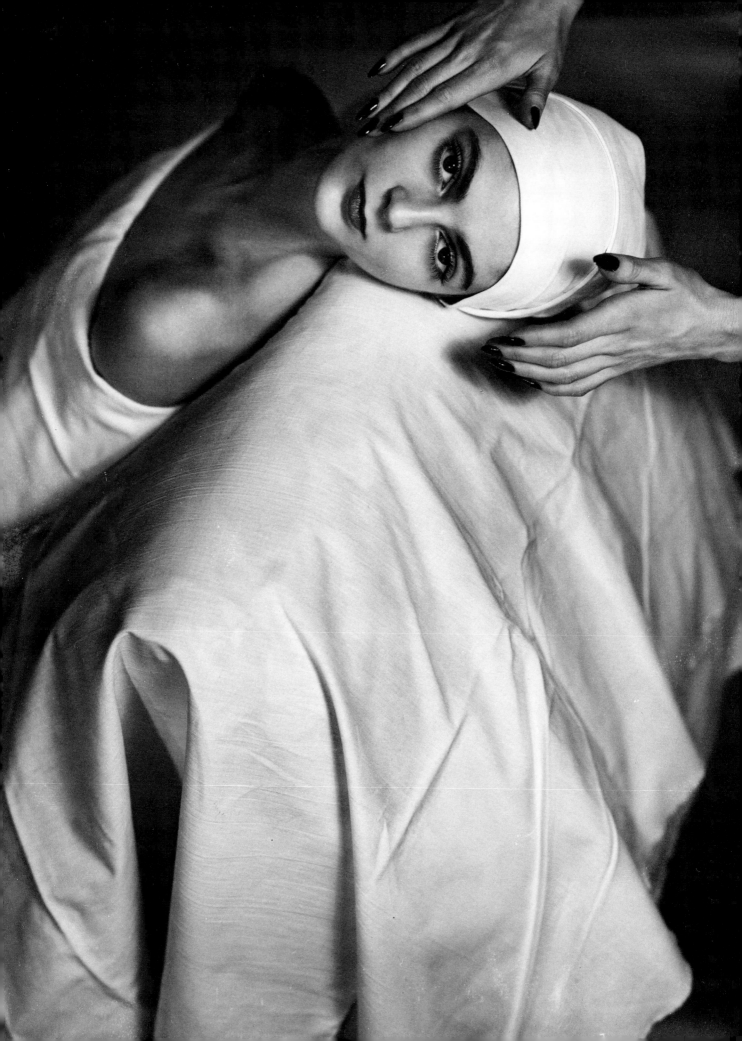

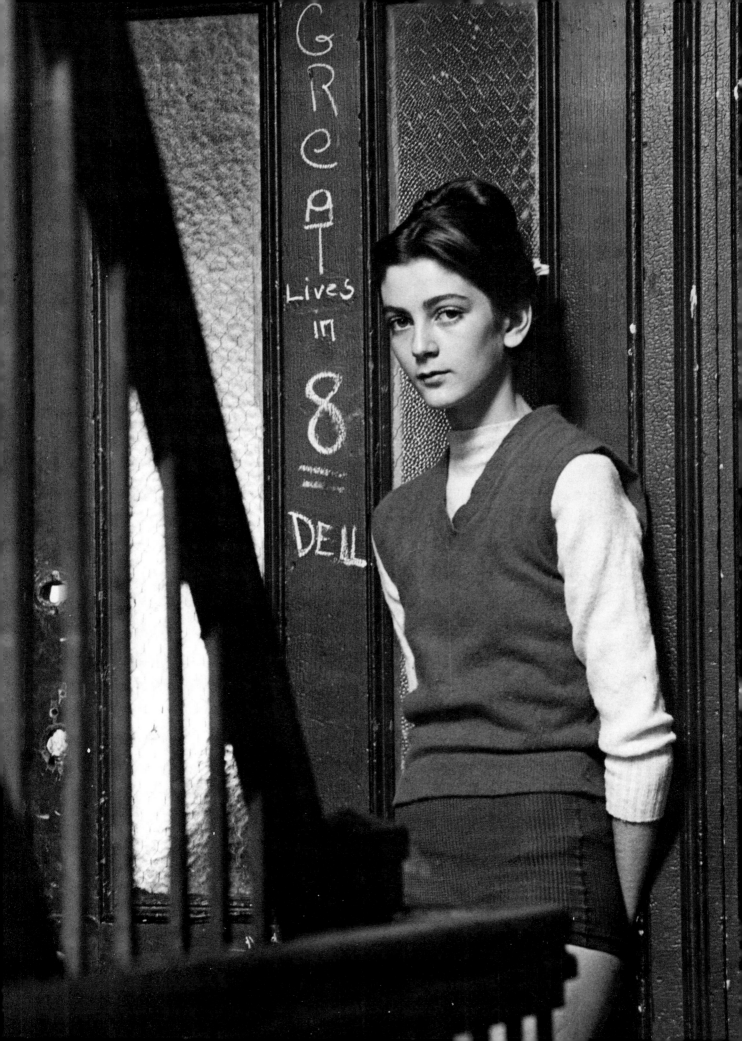

queen of the horsey set, Mrs. John Heminway. Horst selected me. He wrote:

Little Carmen is the ideal painter's beauty; although a sixteen-year-old school girl, she possesses an inherent gracefulness rarely found except among primitive races. Her almond-shaped eyes are those of a Renaissance beauty, a soft revelation when looking up—she tends to keep her well-defined eyelids cast down over them. The planes of her face are those of a Botticelli page, her long neck that of Botticelli's figure of Spring. Her hands are long, aristocratic, and she always manages to keep her shoulders straight. Although she is extremely thin, she is not in the least angular, and moves slowly, softly like an animal. She has two primary requisites of true elegance: the physical attributes of youth and the languor of the past. She is an American beauty of an antique other age.

It was pretty heady stuff, and I was actually only fifteen at the time, but who's counting anymore? Beneath Horst's paean, the editor felt compelled to add her little blurb that reduced the whole thing to the level of winning a Miss Subways contest: "Already a contradiction in glamour and practicality, she cooks, sews, paints, spends long hours at the ballet bar."

Reading Horst's glowing words, one might have thought that my life had changed. Happily, it had not. I say "happily" because I *was* happy, in a constant state of excitement, somehow finding time to do all the things I loved. In that sense, the editor's blurb was truer of me than Horst's tribute, which was more to the image he projected than to the real girl, who was still a normal adolescent trying on a range of activities for size.

I was taking art lessons. The swimming continued. It had become a part of my life that I have

I was already working for Condé Nast when Frances McLaughlin took this picture of me outside the door of the Third Avenue apartment (which had no locks). I did a lot of advertising for myself in chalk. *(Condé Nast)*

not relinquished to this day. It is the world's best exercise. I still went to ballet class. I couldn't bear to give it up, although it was a no-win situation. I had grown too tall, and the muscles developed in swimming were the wrong ones for a dancer. Modeling was the icing on the cake. I loved it and still do. I loved the people I met in the business as I would come to love the world it would eventually open to me. A world I did not yet know in 1946.

We continued to live in the tenement flat above the el, the trains rattling by and setting off seismographically measurable tremors in the apartment. We still did not have a telephone. All of the money I was earning went into my teeth, lessons, and tuition at Lodge, the professional school in which my mother had enrolled me so that I would have time for all my other activities. Away from the cameras, I still looked like some gangling concentration-camp victim fleeing from my captors on roller skates. The gaunt exterior disquieted the great photographer Penn as it did many people. There was no way to tell from my frame that I had developed some formidable long and lithe athlete's muscles between the skin and bones that seemed to cling so closely to each other.

Penn was about to embark on a wonderful series of fairy-tale pictures involving some of the great celebrities of the day and one central figure playing the title roles of Cinderella, Snow White, and Little Red Riding Hood. I longed to be chosen for the job—and not because of the famous supporting cast; Jose Ferrer, Dorothy Parker, Ray Bolger, and the rest were names that meant next to nothing to me. I wanted it because it would give me the chance to be what I was, a young girl, instead of what they called me, "timeless," whatever that was supposed to mean. My time was adolescence, and I was enjoying it too much to want to give it up.

Penn wanted to use me but was worried that I might not have the stamina to hold up through the rigorous shoot. Penn's sessions were always exhausting. He was a great artist, constantly looking for ways to expand the limitations of

21

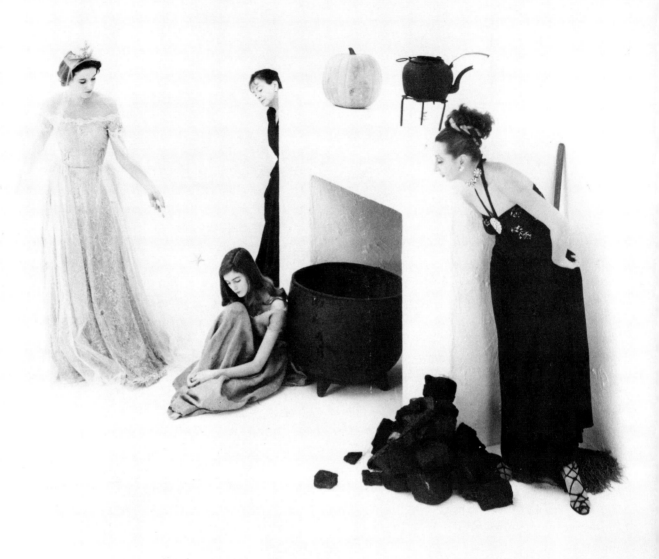

Cinderella from the Penn fairy-tale series. *Left to right:* Mrs. William ("Babe") Paley as the Fairy Godmother; Carmen as Cinderella; Dorothy Parker and Paula Lawrence as the Wicked Stepsisters. *(Irving Penn)*

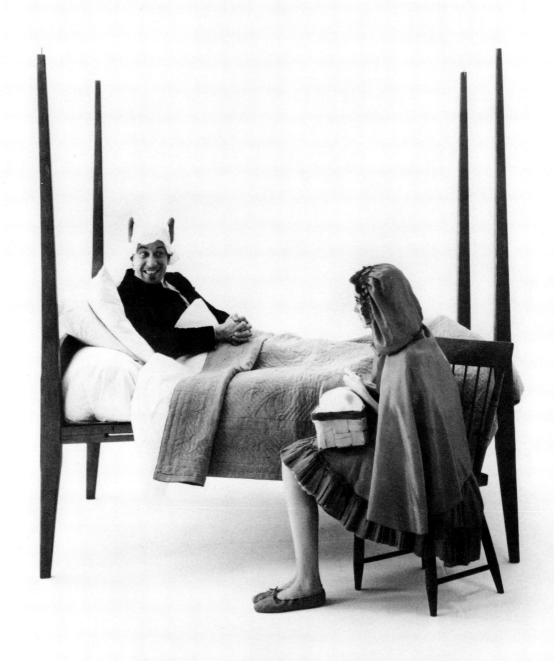

Little Red Riding Hood from the Penn fairy-tale series, with Jose Ferrer as the Wolf. *(Irving Penn)*

film and camera. He once had me hold a single pose for two hours while he experimented with one slow exposure.

I was five-foot-seven and weighed eighty-five pounds. Penn expressed his fears about "little" Carmen's health and insisted I see a doctor before we started to work. An appointment was set up with Dr. Herbert Ogden, the medical supervisor for Condé Nast publications. I had a history of childhood illnesses, most notably the rheumatic fever. From the outside, I may have been *Vogue*'s baby star, the darling of some of the world's most celebrated photographers, but inside I was a mess. Not only was I extremely anemic, I was also prepubescent. I must add that in young ballerinas the latter was not at all unusual. Something in the physical exertion often retarded menstruation.

Dr. Ogden explained to my mother that the real problem was accelerating the maturing process and getting me into puberty. For the anemia he prescribed a vitamin B complex, liver, and iron shots. To speed me into the menstrual cycle, he wanted to try injections of the estrogenic hormones. Estrogen was a new and seldom used treatment for my problem. In the mid-Forties, it was usually administered at the other end of a woman's fertility cycle for menopausal and ovarian cycle complaints. He admitted this was not the normal treatment, but he was convinced it would help me. It was another "scholarship," and mama agreed.

Though I did not have my first period until I was well into my sixteenth year and had nothing that could remotely be described as a bosom until I was seventeen, there were signs that the treatments were working. There was a marked improvement in my blood count and I was gaining weight. When I reached the hundred-pound mark, we had a big celebration.

Dr. and Mrs. Ogden took mama and me under their wing. The four of us would often have dinner together at the Stouffer's restaurant that used to be on Fifty-seventh Street. Another new friend of the period was a young photographer in the *Vogue* studio, Emerick Bronson. He started to photograph me when I was fourteen and hasn't stopped for over forty years, right up to and including many of the pictures in this book. Modeling was indeed changing my life, as dancing had before it. I was beginning to have a circle of friends who appreciated me for what I was. They may all have been adults, but that didn't matter. They were rain after a long drought, and I blossomed and grew.

It may have been because of the shots that were speeding me into adulthood, but another feature began to grow in addition to those I so fervently wished to grow. My nose. It had never been properly attended to after I broke it as a child, and the cartilage went a little crazy, expanding in its own haphazard way. Later, we had it fixed but, at the time, I was a kid with silver bands on every tooth and rubber bands holding my mouth closed and a visibly broken nose. But a loving photographer and brilliant lighting can work wonders, and despite my physical handicaps, I was on my way to being one of the most successful models in town. *Vogue* had upped my pay to $10 an hour, and I was allowed to do outside commercial work. The top advertising rate was then $25 an hour, and only Dorian Leigh, Lisa Fonnsegrives, and I were getting it.

I had more work than I could use, but I was never a great cover girl. My first *Vogue* cover was in October 1947, and I'll never forget the day it came out. I rushed over to a newsstand. There was a stack of magazines on the sidewalk with my picture on the top. I was appalled, hated the way I looked. Oh, I thought, this is the worst thing that can happen! Inside of me, there was this round person fighting to get out, yet on the cover I thought I looked like a boy. I knew better, but compulsively went through the whole pile of magazines hoping to find one picture that looked more like my own image of myself. I was totally crushed when, unsurprisingly, all the covers were the same.

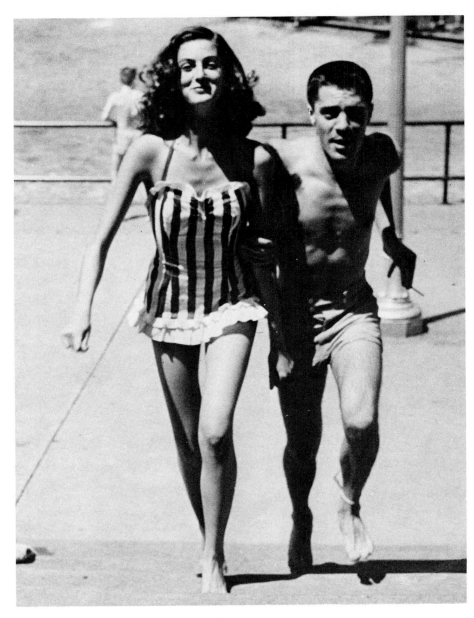

With Emerick Bronson at Jones Beach.

Blumenfeld took that photograph and had to fight with the editors to persuade them to use it. The hint of nudity in a photograph of a sixteen-year-old girl was considered too daring for 1947. It was only after Blumenfeld threatened never to work for Condé Nast again that they reluctantly allowed the cover to run.

Time has proved that the photographer was right. That photo is among the most widely reproduced examples of his work. Critics have expounded on the hint of antiquity and suggestion of narcissism. It will never be among my favorite pictures, but that isn't important. The model is only the subject that reflects the artist's image, and that image is and must be the thing of greatest consequence in a work of art. Our audience is not moved by our work, as they might be by the performance of an actress. They are moved by the picture, and the picture belongs to the photographer.

It must be clear by now that I love my work, and that a good model makes an important con-

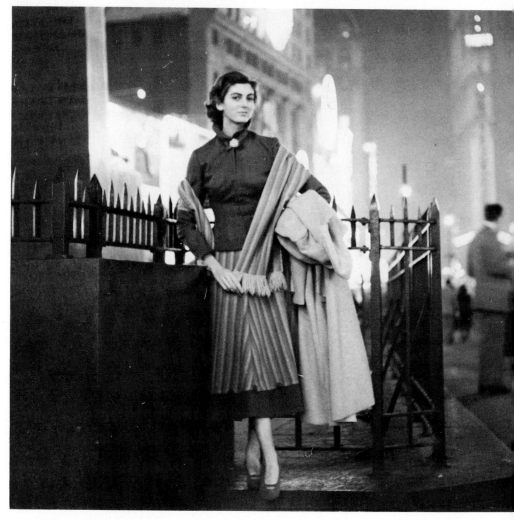

The Bronson photograph that *Vogue* would not use. Nice girls did not stand around Times Square at night.

tribution to the picture by knowing how to give a photographer what he is seeking. But I find the current cult of the model baffling. The camera loves us, the film captures us, but the only thing that may occasionally immortalize us is the art of a Parkinson, or Penn, or Scavullo, or Beaton, or Avedon, or Skrebnesky.

In a great picture, there is an emotional communication between subject and artist that transcends mere prettiness. It is a result of those rare instances when a photographer and model meet in their work and something magical happens. I have been fortunate that this has happened occasionally with several photographers. But it has happened consistently with only one, and that one is Norman Parkinson.

Parkinson is British, and in the Forties most of his work was for English *Vogue* and in European locations, but he occasionally came to New York to do a sitting for the American edition. I first met him when the magazine booked me for a shoot with him in the Hotel Plaza ballroom. It was just another job. His name was unfamiliar, and so I did not react one way or the other and certainly had no inkling of the profound effect he was to have on my career and on my life.

My first *Vogue* cover. How I hated the way I looked! *(Irwin Blumenfeld)*

26

VOGUE

In this issue:
New Kind
of Beauty

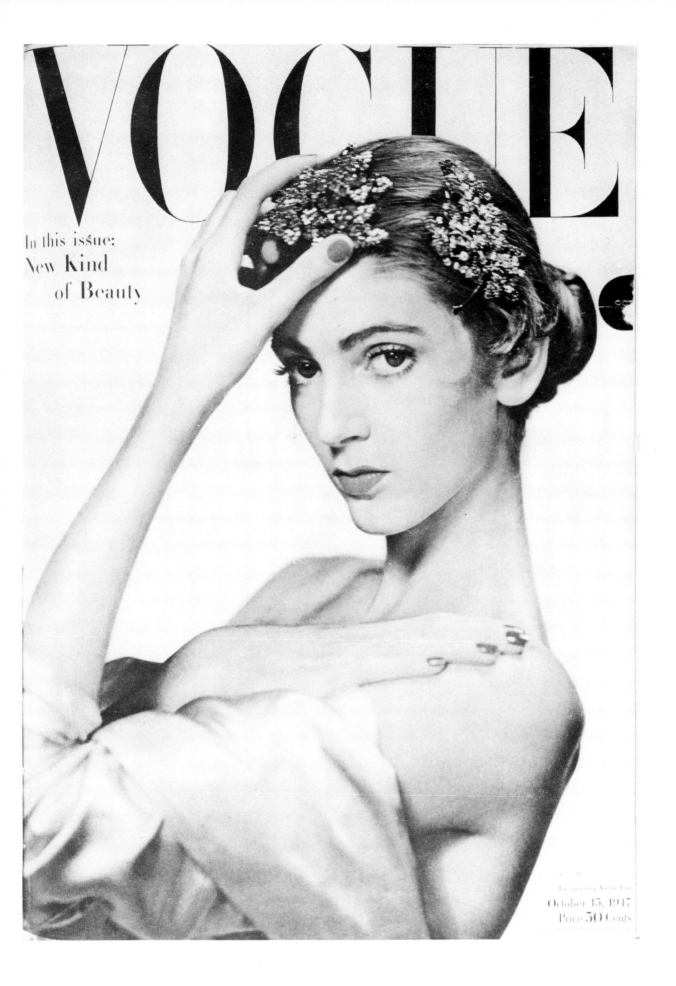

Incorporating Vanity Fair

October 15, 1947
Price 50 Cents

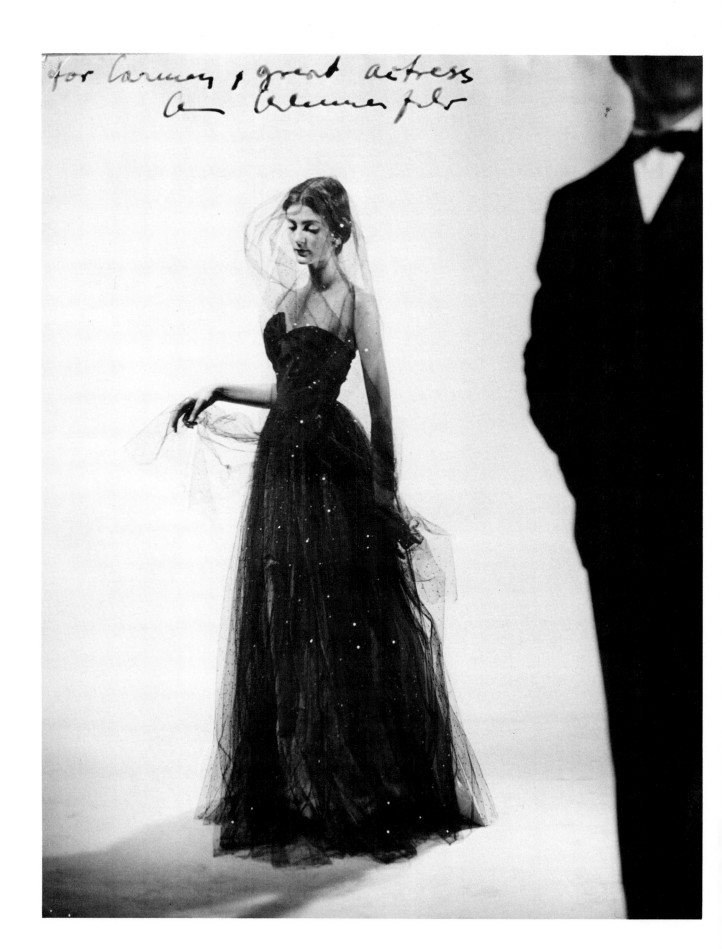

for Carmen, great actress
[signature]

I recall that I was wearing a strapless gray taffeta dress. By then, I had developed just enough of a bosom to carry it without any tissue-paper aids to nature. The fashion editor Bettina Ballard and I were sitting in the ballroom balcony waiting for the photographer. The doors parted and in strolled all six feet six inches of Norman Parkinson. My first reaction was, He's so wonderfully tall. My second reaction was, He's so gorgeous. My third reaction was, I'm in love. I was sixteen and still in my great crush period. Throughout this thrilling first shoot, my heart was going thump, thump, thump. But I don't think it was only adolescent passion that made the work so exciting. My heart has long since stopped thumping at the sight of him, but every time we work together, it is still a great challenge.

"Parks" was and is exacting, patient, witty, temperamental, and eccentric. He can be a pussycat or a lion in his pursuit of what he wants. The important thing is that he has always known what he wants and how to reach that inner core that could draw it out of me. I've been described as having a romantic image, of projecting mystery, allure, a dichotomous combination of distant glamour and grand passion. All of this was first captured on film by Parks. In the beginning, it was my fantasies that he brought to the surface; in our later work, it was my memories—yes, and my regrets. He has this glorious gift for welding my mood to the ambience in which we are working, be it Newport, or San Simeon, or Paris, or some remote tropical beach, or swinging dizzily above London on a building crane, which he once had me do for a British cover. The point is that we trust each other professionally and, trusting each other, we take chances.

With that first Plaza shoot, I lost all shyness

as a model, which was remarkable because at the time I was almost self-effacing with other photographers. It was an instant rapport, a sparking off each other—I dared, and he double-dared.

By the end of the day, my fluttery heart had confused professional passion with emotional passion, and I was having visions of this perfect relationship. And then the doors to the ballroom opened again to admit the most beautiful woman I had ever seen, with an enchanting three-year-old boy in tow. I was introduced to Parks's wife, Wenda, and his son, Simon. My fluttery heart went whacko!

Private passions spent, the professional passion has survived. Through all the years, no matter what emotional shape I was in, what physical size I was, what color my hair was (and it's been every color of the rainbow at one time or another), Parkinson would book me sight unseen from Europe or Tobago, where he and Wenda live. A cable or a letter would arrive— "Pack your things, we've got a location at the other end of the world" or "Book out of everything else the week after next"—and I was ready. How often, at my lowest periods, I've searched the mail for that wonderful scrawl of his on an envelope, and how often he intuitively knew that I needed a lift and he was there to supply it.

II

A year later, I was on the cover of the November 1, 1948, issue of *Vogue* in a photograph taken by Rawlings. My face was wrapped in veiling, my body in broadtail and sable. I was leaning suggestively toward a man just out of camera range. I was seventeen going on thirty-five and looked it. The inside copy read: "For a man's eye (there could be a gleam in it), a woman who looks as if she would neither simper nor whistle for her own taxi."

I loved the whole idea of the picture. To me,

My favorite Blumenfeld photograph. He inscribed it "For Carmen, great actress." *(Irwin Blumenfeld)*

it was "hot stuff." The year had made a difference, and that difference was men. I still had braces and a broken nose, but everything else about me was changing, and this photograph was how I longed to see myself: sophisticated, soignée, in charge of the situation. By the way, we still lived on Third Avenue, but even Third Avenue was changing. The el was coming down, and another Third Avenue girl, by the name of Bobo, was marrying a Rockefeller.

Dr. Ogden's treatments had worked, and I came of sexual age during the long twilight of the cult of the virgin, which coincided with the post–World War II baby boom. Don't ask me how men managed both at the same time, I still don't know. As far as girls were concerned, we didn't know which was more difficult or important—losing our virginity or keeping it. One thing is certain, we did a lot of worrying about it, which is more than my daughter's generation did, or less, depending on your point of view. Let's call it "progress" and not attempt to analyze in which direction.

There was a lot of sexual tension around, which made both men and women act most peculiarly. We had all of the same desires and physical needs as girls of today, but we rarely if ever did anything about it. During the late Forties, there was all this unchanneled energy in the air. We wanted to be near, to touch, but we didn't know how near or what should be touched. We had dozens of shibboleths about "good girls" and "bad girls," about kissing with the mouth open and kissing with the mouth closed, about petting above the waist and petting below the waist, and about how far to go on the first, second, and third dates. There were so many rules that one was tempted to stay home with a good book. The only problem was the primary rule, which was, on pain of death, never be without a date on Saturday night.

Emotions were closer to the surface because passions were so inhibited. We cried and laughed and felt everything so much more deeply because we needed a release for frustrations we could not name. Everything had to be

The first picture taken of me for *Vogue* by Norman Parkinson. That's all Carmen and not tissue paper holding the dress up. Thank you very much, Dr. Ogden. *(Norman Parkinson)*

romantic, and filled with illusion, and beautiful. The music to which we danced held us close. We did not want the songs to end, because of the intimate contact of faces and bodies. In those days, there were no soloists doing their own things out there on the floor, and strobe lights were in the far future; our lighting was as dim and flattering as candles. The places we frequented were elegant, with none of the contemporary brutality of enameled walls and exposed steel beams. Ankle-length circular skirts —Dior's "new look"—had just come in. Insiders knew all that fabric was being used because Dior was owned by a fabric company that wanted to sell its wares. To us, however, the clothes evoked a distant romantic era and mirrored our own feelings. There was time for romance, and we had all of that pent-up energy with which to ardently pursue it.

I came of age in that era, and my professional image was shaped by it. It pleases and suits me. I love romance and still cannot think of physical intimacy without it. I was naïve, and in many ways am still naïve. There are many things that I consciously choose not to know. If it makes me old-fashioned, then old-fashioned is my style and signature and I'll happily stick with it. The essence of romance and illusion is actually "Less is more."

The recent resurgence of my career and call for my look would seem to indicate that romance is making a comeback. When I think about it, the mid-Eighties in New York City are not unlike the late Forties. Restaurants are getting lush again even if what they serve is a variation on lean cuisine. Night life abounds, and young people are again extremely fashion-conscious. Getting into the "best" places is now, as it was then, a hassle with headwaiters

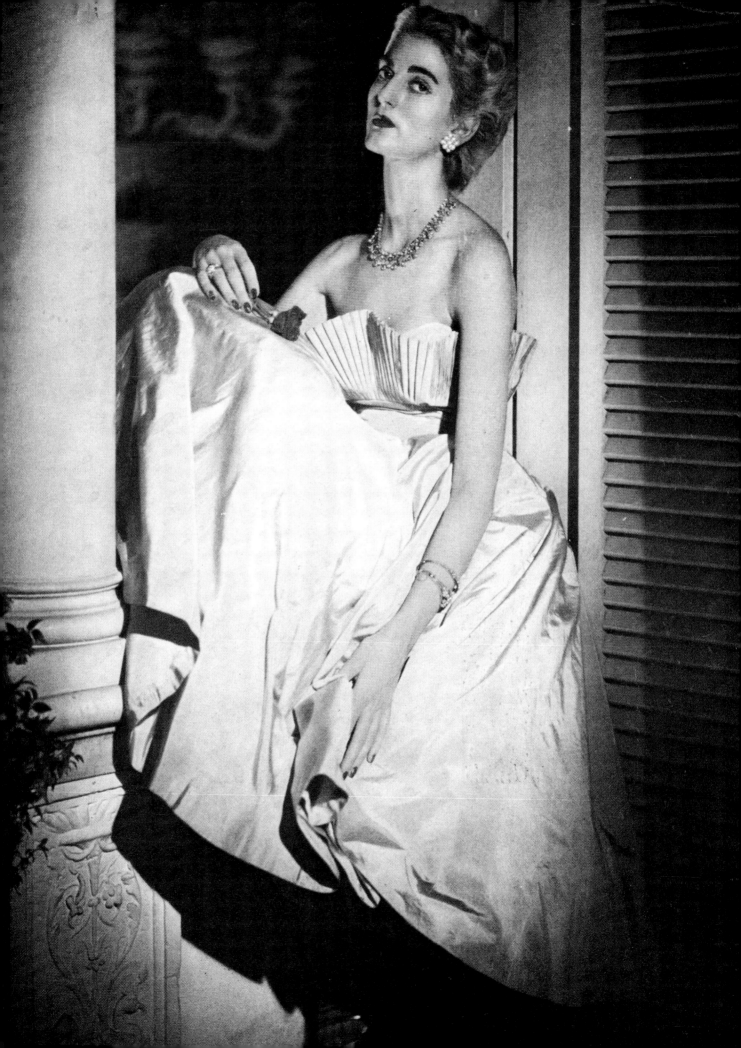

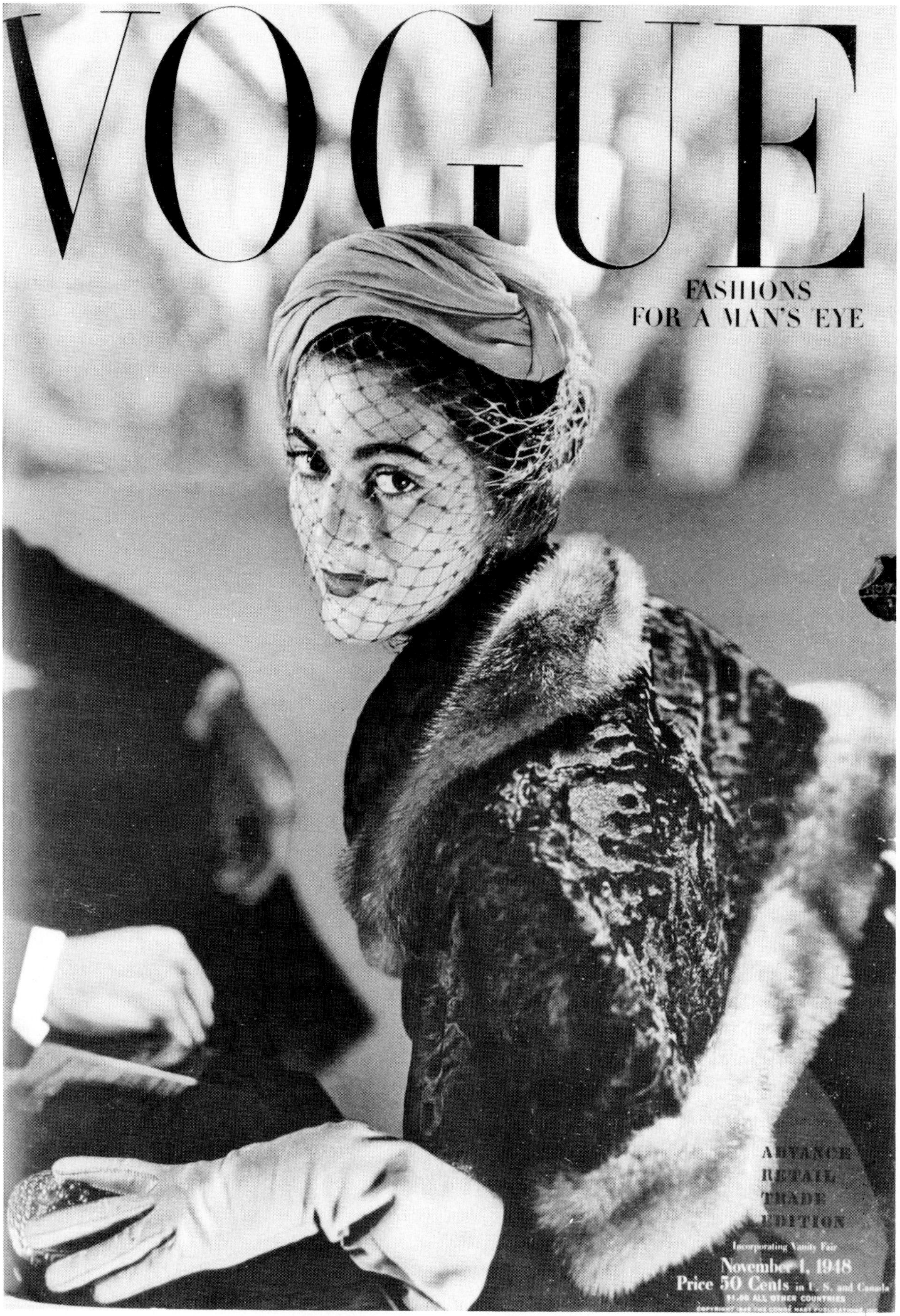

VOGUE

FASHIONS
FOR A MAN'S EYE

ADVANCE
RETAIL
TRADE
EDITION

Incorporating Vanity Fair
November 1, 1948
Price 50 Cents in U. S. and Canada
$1.00 ALL OTHER COUNTRIES
COPYRIGHT 1948 THE CONDÉ NAST PUBLICATIONS INC.

unless you are well known, well dressed, well heeled, or, best of all, some marvelous combination of the three. More champagne and less cocaine is being consumed at the better parties. Dancing cheek-to-cheek is making a comeback. Singles bars are considered about as square as a cube. Best of all, people are taking the time to court. They are holding out for commitment as a part of concupiscence. I am again beginning to feel very much at home in my own time. In the Sixties, somebody once flippantly said to me, "Don't worry, darling, your type will come back."

Looking back and ahead, I think it has!

In my youth, I made my first acquaintance with the innest night spot, El Morocco, a few years before I even knew what it was. In those days, the club was located just around the corner from where we lived. I was fourteen and had just begun to work for *Vogue,* but I was still "walking" Honey on my roller skates. I've always been a scavenger (I still prowl around looking for pieces of furniture people throw out that can be made serviceable again with just a little tender loving care) and my youthful hunting took me to a nearby garbage pail on Fifty-fourth Street that had the most succulent bones for Honey. One day when I went on my hunt, there was a forbidding-looking man in dinner clothes chomping on a cigar and pacing back and forth on the pavement with his hands folded behind his back. I was churning through the pail when he shouted, "What do you think you're doing, little girl? Get your hands out of that muck!"

He asked where I lived and insisted on taking me home and coming up all four flights. My mother was at home at the time and explained that she knew I went through the trash looking for bones for the dog. She added indignantly that we were not so poor we ate other people's garbage. He kept insisting it was not the proper thing for a young lady to be doing. He said, "I'll tell you what. You get her to quit it and I'll see there's a good bag of bones left for her every day."

The man was John Perona, and he owned El Morocco. Some people thought he was a thug; others thought him a great character; but I've always thought he was a lovely gentleman. When he heard that our name was Dell'Orefice, he assumed we were Italian and became our friend. He even had my mother to the club for dinner. When I started dating, El Morocco was one of the places to which I was taken, and he always kept a watchful eye on me. I may have been longing for a man to make a pass, but hands always remained above the table when Mr. Perona was around. As for those bags of bones, they often contained thick, juicy steaks fresh from the kitchen and definitely not intended for Honey.

Men as potential mates, or dates, or fates, or hates, or even swinging gates, did not become a part of my life until a few years after my first encounter with Mr. Perona. I was sixteen and had become the favorite model of Mr. John, the famous hat designer. Calling him a "milliner" or "hatmaker" would not do justice to what he did; "confectioner" would be closer to the mark. His hats were fantasies of tulle lace, feathers, veiling, and flowers. One has to recall the Forties to know what a hat can mean to a woman. It was essential, her crowning glory, and often could cost more than the suit or dress it was meant to accessorize. An Easter bonnet was worthy of the wonderful song Mr. Berlin wrote about it, and on Easter Sunday all of the great hat designers of the period would gather their favorite models, adorn them with these marvelous structures, and parade them on Fifth Avenue, which in those days was awash with the essence of feminine frivolity.

Mr. John courted a resemblance to Napoleon in both looks and behavior. He was an autocrat, but often an adorable autocrat, and in my six-

My second *Vogue* cover. I loved it. I was 17 and looked 35. *(John Rawlings)*

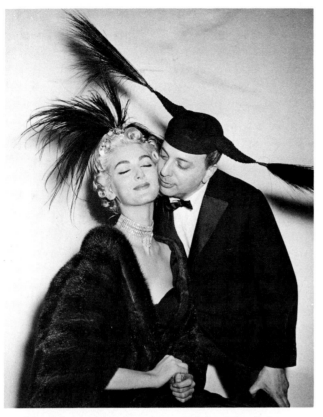

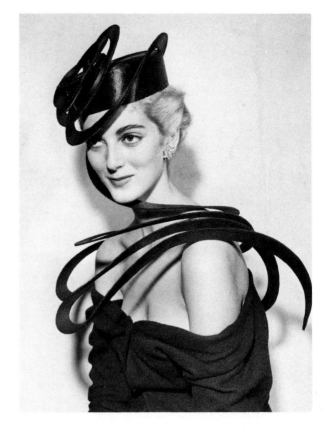

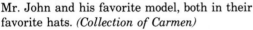
Mr. John and his favorite model, both in their favorite hats. *(Collection of Carmen)*

teenth year his salon became one of my regular stops along Fifty-seventh Street. When I was working there one day, my mother came along for some reason. It may have been to pick up fabric—he was always giving us the ends of bolts, from which we made our party clothes. At any rate, that day he took her aside and said that he felt I was living much too confined an existence—classes, work, and nothing more. It was time I broadened my horizon to include men. He said, "I will give a party for Carmen and invite all of the eligible young bachelors. She will be launched."

When Mr. John said he was going to do something, nobody, not even mama, dared to contradict. It was a splendid party, about twenty men and me. Some of them were not all that young, and all were older than me, but they were wonderful. I was the deliriously happy but still unsmiling girl of the moment. Many of

them asked me for dates, and it was then that they came up against mama's one condition before allowing the party: If they wanted to take me out, these worldly-wise fellows first had to submit to an old-world interview conducted by my suspicious mother. Nobody objected. I think it was all that virginity business. Everybody put such a high store on it that these men could understand a mother's concern before entrusting her daughter's precious jewel to them. I discovered later that there was another reason. In the circles in which these gents traveled even back then, there was not that much virginity around. It was getting so scarce that it topped the list of endangered species. The hunters were caught in a no-man's-land, trapped between a desire to use up the available supply and a feeling of moral allegiance to some sort of sexual conservationism.

Pat DeCicco was among the men to whom

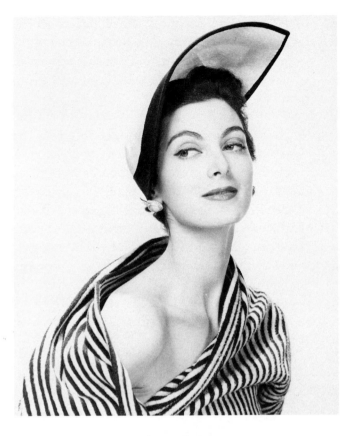
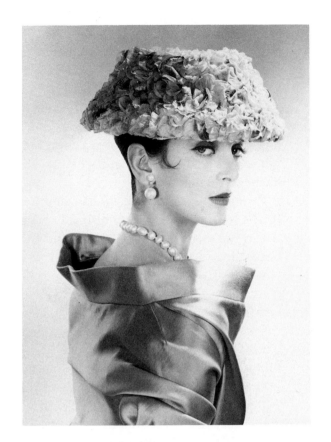
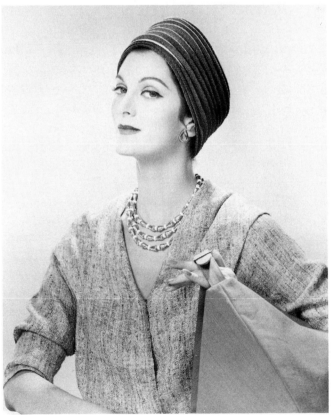
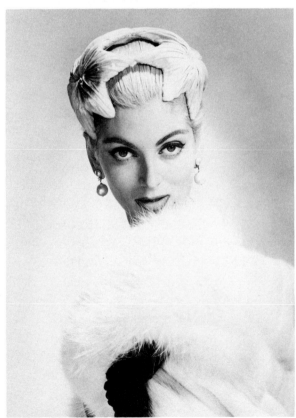

Mr. John introduced me. He was closer to my mother's age than mine and was known as "the broccoli king of Long Island." Lest you get the idea he was a farmer, let me assure you that what Pat plowed bore no relationship to a field of vegetables. He was one of our leading lady-killers and presumably did for Gloria Vanderbilt what he never did for me when he was her husband number one.

Pat was my first grown-up date and inevitably he took me to our local bistro, El Morocco. It was the first time I'd gotten beyond the garbage cans. I was wearing a beautiful black taffeta dress I'd made from fabric Mr. John had given to me. It was about eight in the evening, late for me but early for El Morocco, although there was a fairly large dinner crowd in attendance. John Perona was at the door, and when I appeared, he completely lost the kingly cool with which he managed his place, regally designating who might or might not be permitted to enter. He began to sputter at Pat that he could not bring this child into a nightclub. He turned to me and sternly asked if my mother knew where I was and with whom.

I tried to reassure him that I had mama's permission, but he would not accept my word for it. We still had no telephone. Telling us to wait right there, Perona ran around the corner and up those four flights to speak to my mother. He demanded to know if she was aware that her daughter was in his place with an infamous playboy.

With a combination of Latin charm and subliminal flirtation, Pat had passed mama's screening. She told Perona she knew all about it. She said, "Mr. DeCicco and I are friends. He's promised to bring Carmen home right after dinner."

A chastened Perona returned and allowed us to join the table of a couple with whom Pat had made an engagement. Pat told me that I could have anything I wanted, and so I ordered shrimp, a steak, and a "snowball," a sinfully delectable vanilla-ice-cream concoction with hot fudge and coconut. When I finished, he asked if I was happy and had had enough. I replied that I was happy but not full, and asked if I could start again. He said, "You mean with another snowball?"

"No. With the shrimp."

He replied that it was all right with him, if I was sure I could finish another complete meal. I said I was and proceeded to prove it. In those days, I had that kind of appetite because I was expending so much energy at swimming, ballet, and work. I never ate between meals, but I certainly made up for it at them. I was developing good habits among the bad ones. Although today I would not dream of eating the quantity I put away in those days, I've still got a healthy appetite and, more important, I still don't eat between meals.

Igor Cassini was another man to whom Mr. John introduced me. One day, Igor called mama and asked if he might take me to lunch with a gentleman who had seen and admired me at El Morocco. He assured her that the man could be very helpful to me; and mama, assuming he meant helpful with my career, allowed me to go. I was barely sixteen, and the gentleman to whom Igor introduced me was not only older but so much older that I immediately thought of him as a sweet and harmless grandfatherly type. Our lunch took place in a wonderful and truly elegant French restaurant, Chambord, a few blocks south of our home on Third Avenue. (The el shaded not only the tenement homes of the poor but also some of the favorite watering holes of the rich.) For dessert, we had one of the light-as-air soufflés for which Chambord was famous. As I look back, those early dates were far more memorable for the meals I ate than for the men with whom I ate them.

After lunch, the gentleman and Gigi (Igor's nickname) and I went for a stroll on Park Avenue. In those days, Park Avenue in the fifties was lined with luxurious apartment buildings. At the entrance to one of them, the gentleman

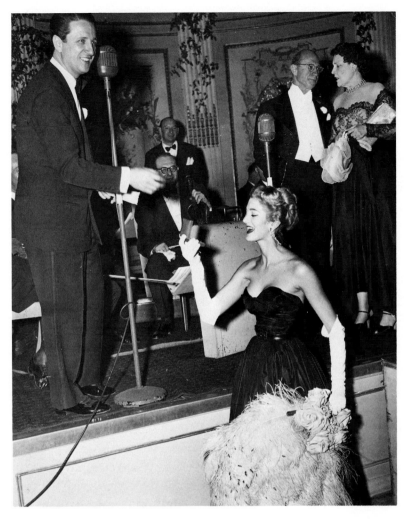

The columnist Cholly (Igor Cassini) Knickerbocker presenting an award to me in the early 1950s. I made the dress myself; décolletage wasn't usually so plunging at that time. A few years before, Cholly had wanted to make another kind of presentation. *(Collection of Carmen)*

asked if I'd like to come up and see his place. I must explain that Cassini was better known as Cholly Knickerbocker, the nationally syndicated gossip columnist. I like Gigi very much and prefer to believe that the introduction was made in all innocence. As I've said, I thought of the older man as quite harmless and sweet, and so I had no qualms about going with him.

The paintings and antique furniture and even the wall-to-wall carpeting were overwhelming to a girl from Third Avenue. The man asked if mama and I would like to live there. I replied that it was so beautiful I knew my mother would love to live in it, and he told me to go home and ask her, because he would love to have us as his guests.

I raced home and told mama that we were moving. I suppose mama was trying to help me get on in the world, and help herself in the process, but this was too much. She was not about to let me move in with Joseph P. Kennedy. When we later reminisced about the event, she said with a sigh, "If he only wanted to introduce you to one of his sons, that would have been a different story."

I had become one of those well-known faces that well-known names liked to be seen with, and I began to go out with some rather racy members of what was then called "café society." I had turned seventeen in June 1948. During that summer, I was part of many weekend parties at the Port of Missing Men, Peter Salm's house in Southampton, which was then the Hamptons' headquarters for all of the better-known young men around town. I was on my way out for my very first weekend there when I met a man who would change my life.

Peter picked me up late on a Friday afternoon, and to avoid traffic we stopped off at a cocktail party at a friend's home on Fifth Avenue. I was sitting off to one side by myself watching the others dance, thinking it had to be the handsomest, gayest, wittiest crowd in the world, and that only by some minor miracle had I become part of it. I watched a very good-looking man, probably in his late twenties, make his way across the room and hoped he was coming toward me. He was. He introduced himself as Bill Miles, sat down beside me, and immediately launched into a tirade on how a child like me had no business going off with a jaded and sophisticated group like the Salm crowd. He warned me about what would happen and described how they would inflict themselves on me. Not even my mother had ever painted such a graphic portrait of "the fate worse than death."

That over with, he abruptly asked me to dance. Would you believe that, for all my ballet training, I didn't know how to fox-trot? It was true. He pulled me to my feet and said he would teach me—and he did. I was very taken with Mr. William Miles and so shy that I barely spoke ten words, which was fine with him, because he enjoyed doing all the talking. I prayed that he would call me when I got back to town (yes, by then, we finally did have a phone), but it was almost a month before he got around to it.

For all of Bill's warnings, nothing happened that weekend nor on any of the subsequent weekends at the Port of Missing Men. They treated me like a kid sister. When the conversation rolled around to sex, my innocence shone like a beacon. I would like to think it was respect for that innocence that kept them from

Through the years with Vanity Fair. Ten lovely years at $300 an hour in a campaign that was supposed to end my career. (Richard Avedon)

making advances, but I really know better. What was actually going on were bets on which of them would be the first to bed me down. In their eagerness to win, each was keeping an eagle eye on me to make certain none of the others beat him to the act. They were all so good at the job, there was no act and, so to speak, the bets were the only things that were lost.

Over the years, I've told and retold these stories to friends in roughly the same terms in which I have just set them down. They've become a polished party act—Carmen and Her First Experiences with Men. What amazes me is that it did not occur to me until very recently how small a part my own will played in them. I've dismissed my part in what happened or did not happen with bland excuses such as naïveté, innocence, inexperience. But as a young woman moving through the rarefied world I had entered, what did I really feel? How much did my beloved here-again-gone-again father color my responses to men? Largely, it is almost as if the young me did not exist except as a receptacle for men's desires.

Bill Miles was divorced and had a young son who lived with Bill's ex-wife's parents. He was the first serious romance of my life and perfect for the role. That he was several years older was also right, for I needed a man who could be a combination of teacher/sophisticate/lover. Throughout my adolescence, I had experienced a series of wild crushes, but this was the first man for whom I had ever felt a deep and conscious sexual desire, and I collided with the wall of that Forties virginity attitude. It was our first major problem, but strangely enough the problem was his and not mine. He wanted me as much as I wanted him, but he did not want to

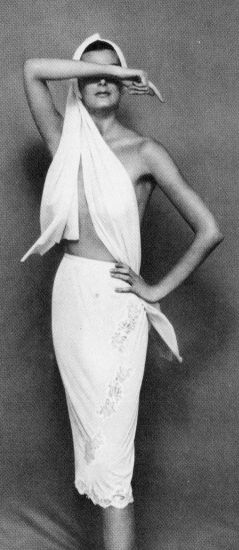

VANITY FAIR

dramatic slant: a discreet diagonal of
our fine Alençon lace, delicately appliqued   on this nylon tricot pettiskirt. 8.95

Vanity Fair Mills, Inc., 640 Fifth Avenue, N.Y.

Richard Avedon

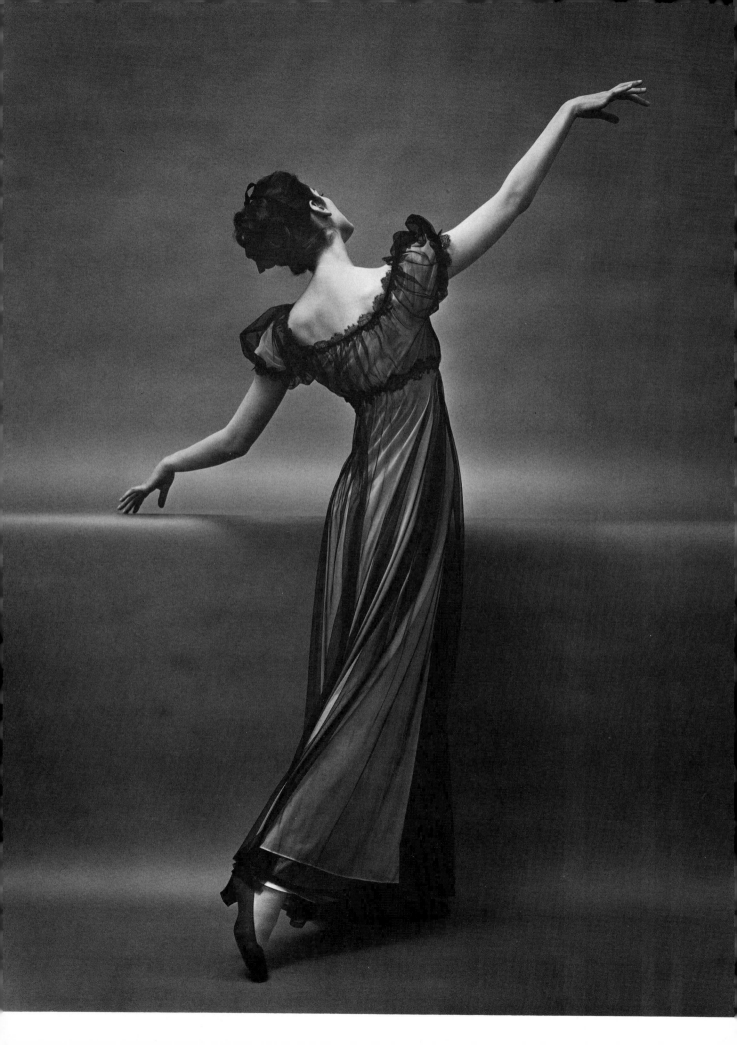

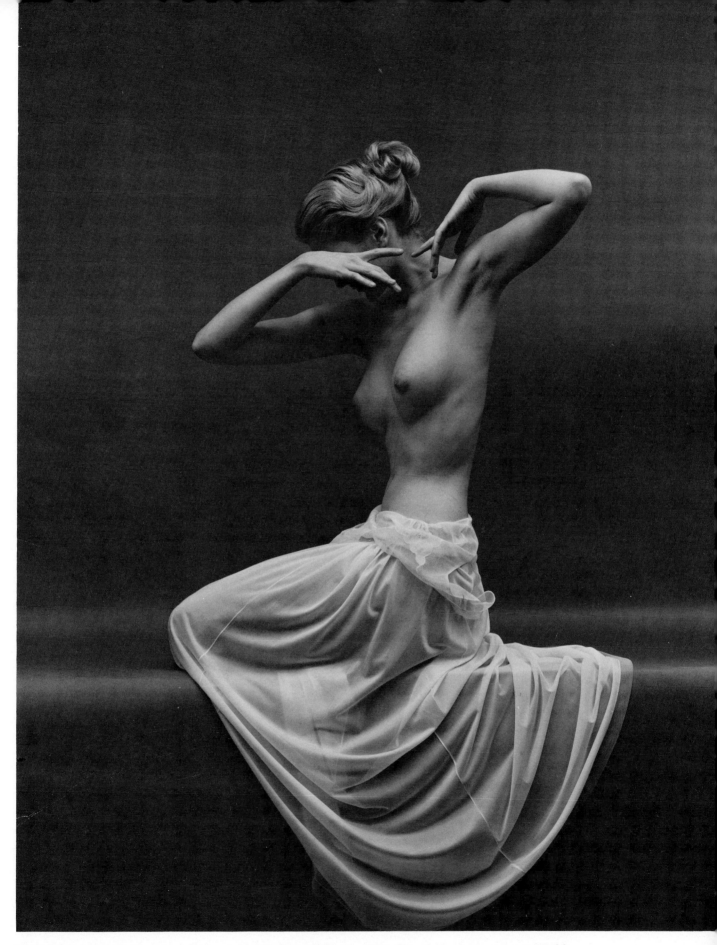

Mark Shaw photographs taken during a Vanity Fair sitting in 1950. The photo above was *not* used by the company. *(Mark Shaw)*

be the first. He did not want the responsibility of going to bed with a virgin, especially when he loved her. If it did not work for me the first time, he did not want to take the chance that it might change what we felt for each other.

It was certainly a unique dilemma, and I solved it in the only possible way. In my eighteenth year, my nose was fixed, my braces were removed, and I lost my virginity. Once those things were attended to, I took a giant leap forward and did what no girl of my age ever did at the time. Bill and I set up housekeeping together, and after a long and successful trial run, we were finally married when I was twenty-one.

Along with the drastic changes in my private life, there was a great alteration in my career. Dr. Ogden's shots had really worked their magic: I had been growing into womanhood and losing the look that first turned me into a successful model. *Vogue*'s baby star had been gradually setting, and there were fewer calls from the magazine for my services. By the time I was eighteen, I had become a full-busted, broad-shouldered amazon and had moved from being too small for a perfect model's size to being too large. My look was all wrong for the time, and even the advertising, which had been so lucrative, was falling off.

If my career ended, so what? thought I. I was in love and did not need it. The typical product of my times, I believed that you found a man, got married, had babies, and became a housewife. I was wrong. I was in love and did need the career. Bill and I were used to a certain life-style, and to maintain it I had to contribute to our income. We were experiencing then what so many young couples experience now.

During those first few years of my career, a new power arose and took control of the business. It was the model agency. At first there were only two of any importance, John Robert Powers and Harry Conover, and I was with Powers. Other agencies began to appear as the

With my new baby, Laura; new nose, and new hair color. *(Collection of Carmen)*

Forties became the Fifties. The new girl in town was Eileen Ford, and when my career began to fade, I decided to try my luck with her. Eileen took one look at my size and said there was absolutely nothing she could do for me.

I eventually went with a lovely woman named Frances Gill who had that rare commodity, sympathy, and did not look upon her models as merely merchandise. Frances said she would do what she could, but did not hold out any high hopes. Unless a miracle happened, my days as a star were over.

Most of the leading models were washed up by the time they were thirty, but twenty seemed a bit extreme. The miracle did happen, however, and my second career began. Frances called to say that Vanity Fair, the well-known lingerie manufacturer, wanted my exclusive services for an advertising campaign ("exclusive" meaning that I would not appear in any other lingerie ads but was free to work at anything else). It was a big job because the line was so extensive and the ads appeared in every slick magazine and newspaper in the country. Nonetheless, Frances suggested I think it over very carefully. It would mean the end of my high-fashion career since there was an unwritten law that "class" models did not pose in their own or anybody else's undies.

All of my friends in the business warned me I would be committing professional suicide, but as far as I was concerned, the fashion phase was just about over anyway, so there was nothing to lose. I called Frances and told her, if the money was right, I would do it.

The money was very right. It was $300 an hour, which for many years made me the highest-paid model in the world. They were willing to go that high to get that very rare bird, a *Vogue* star who had hips and breasts.

What my friends did not understand was

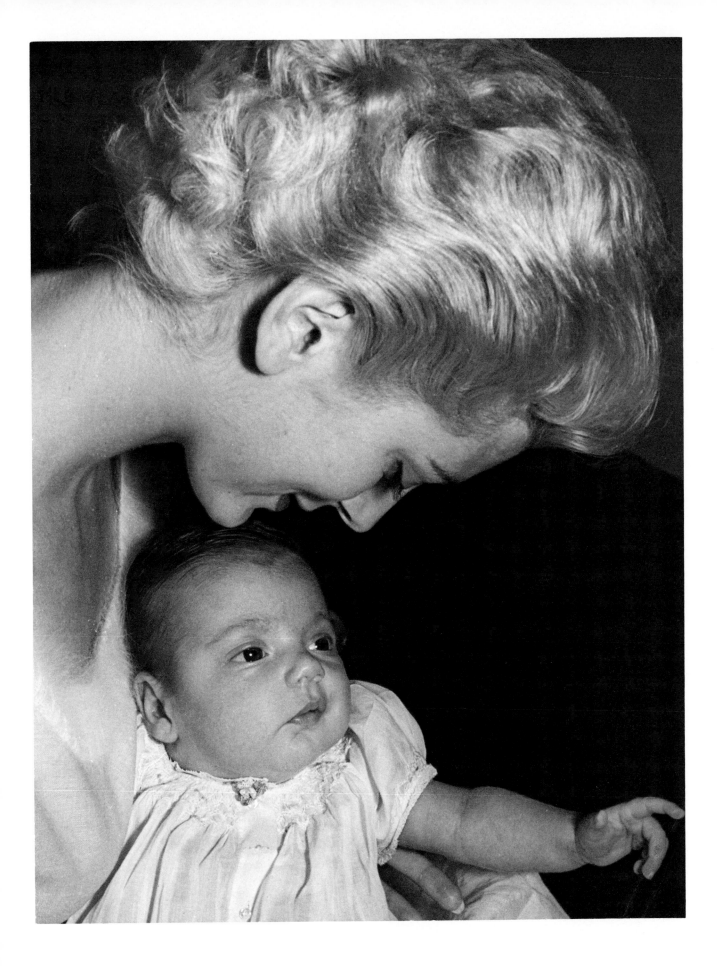

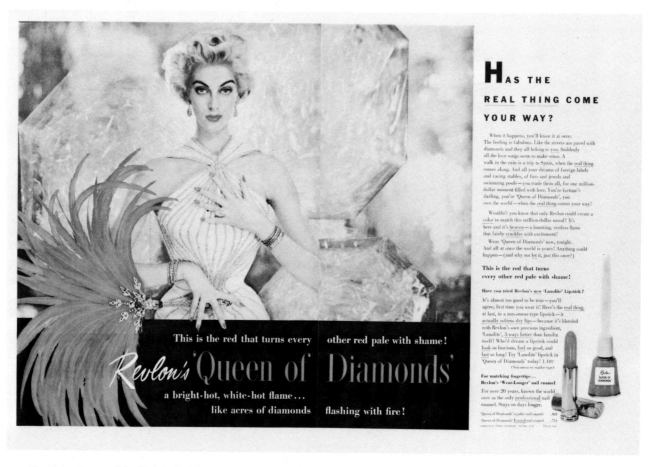

Back to the world of high fashion. One of the most widely distributed Revlon ads spread over two pages in full color. *(Richard Avedon)*

that, from Vanity Fair's prospective, it was a "class" campaign. The concept belonged to Mr. Barbie, the president of Vanity Fair. You could say I was a Barbie doll long before Mattel ever dreamt of the toy that has made millions for them. Mr. Barbie's idea was simplicity itself. The body and the lingerie were the important things. Only the back of my head or a small portion of my face would ever be revealed. I knew what my mother's reaction would be. Even with a new nose and no braces, she would be certain something was terribly wrong, and I had retrogressed to those early days when Clifford Coffin covered my features with a tea cup.

I worked for Vanity Fair for ten years. My hands were raised to my brow so often in those photographs that the inside name for the Van-

ity Fair symbol was "the girl with the Excedrin headache." But they contributed to a change in women's attitudes: We became proud of our figures, took better care of them, and were unashamed of exhibiting them when they were looking their best. Those ads, the bikini bathing suit, the Marilyn Monroe calendar, and the *Playboy* centerfold all happened at about the same time. I might add, somewhat immodestly, that Vanity Fair was considered the class act of the lot. Some have since said our bodies were being exploited by men. But even a great advocate of women's rights like Jane Fonda doesn't seem averse to displaying her body and making a few cents along the way.

Within a few years of the appearance of the first Vanity Fair ads, *Harper's Bazaar* and *Vogue* were featuring their first nude photographs. The "class" models were clamoring to pose in half-slips and bras—and less. The same pals—models and photographers—who had predicted the end of my career were calling to ask if I could get Mr. Barbie to hire them.

Eileen Ford, too, changed her mind and was convinced the time had come for my return to high fashion, and that she was just the woman to manage it. It was 1953, only four years after the worst had been predicted about that part of my career, but she was right. Before I could avail myself of Eileen's services, I had to attend to something else. I was pregnant.

My weight at the onset of my pregnancy was 125 pounds, but by the time my darling Laura was born, I was tipping the scale at 175. I lost only twenty pounds with the birth, and 155 was no weight to start being a fashion star again. My good friend Dorian Leigh took me by the hand and led me to Nicholas Kounovsky's exercise studio. Nicky gave my body back to me in better shape than it had been before my pregnancy—and in the process completely altered the way I thought about fitness.

I had never really exercised. Swimming had been all that was necessary to keep me fit (and it remains the best of all exercises). From the day of the first Kounovsky exercise class, not a day has passed without a small portion of it devoted to stretch exercise and some simple forms of gymnastics. I've been lucky—my career led me to exercise very early on and has kept me at it ever since. But it is never too late for any of us to get in shape. You don't need a career for motivation; all you need is a desire for well-being and balance. Balance and moderation are the keys to a good, and beautiful, and healthy life for all women of my age—indeed, for all women of any age. Much more than men, I think we have to find our center of gravity, our golden mean, and not deviate from it.

It took eighteen months to get down to my normal weight. I had no special diet except avoiding excess. We know what foods are fat-tening. We also know that a certain number of carbohydrates are necessary to good health. There is no need to torture ourselves with the latest diet craze unless there is a real obesity problem, and in that case the family doctor will be far more helpful than any food "mania" from Oxford, Beverly Hills, Cambridge, or Scarsdale. To lose weight, the best diet is common sense. I'm going to repeat the fundamentals: balance and moderation. Excess is the enemy; it will lead us astray in every area of our inner lives as well as in the things we do to our appearances. *Excess* can mean too little as well as too much, and it goes for everything from sex to eye shadow. No matter what you've heard, there *is* such a thing as too thin. For an objective and balanced outlook on life, there can even be such a thing as too rich.

Because I did not crash-diet and had developed a disciplined exercise regime to accompany my commonsense attitude toward food, I have kept the weight off for the thirty years that have passed since Laura's birth. By the way, I kept on doing the Vanity Fair ads even while I was heavy; a peignoir covers a multitude of sins.

It was a different person who looked back from the photographs. I was no longer the ethereal wraith of the early years, nor the pinup who followed. If one could judge by appearances, this was a woman who had acquired a certain amount of worldly wisdom and élan. How fundamental the change was can be measured by what was happening in my private life. Our marriage was disintegrating. To give the reasons would involve a great many recriminations and counterrecriminations that have no place here. Let's simply say I had grown up and away, and that Bill had needs I could no longer satisfy. The fashion world of my youth had brought Bill into my life, but my reentry would have to be alone.

It was a new start with a new magazine. My editorial assignments had switched from *Vogue*

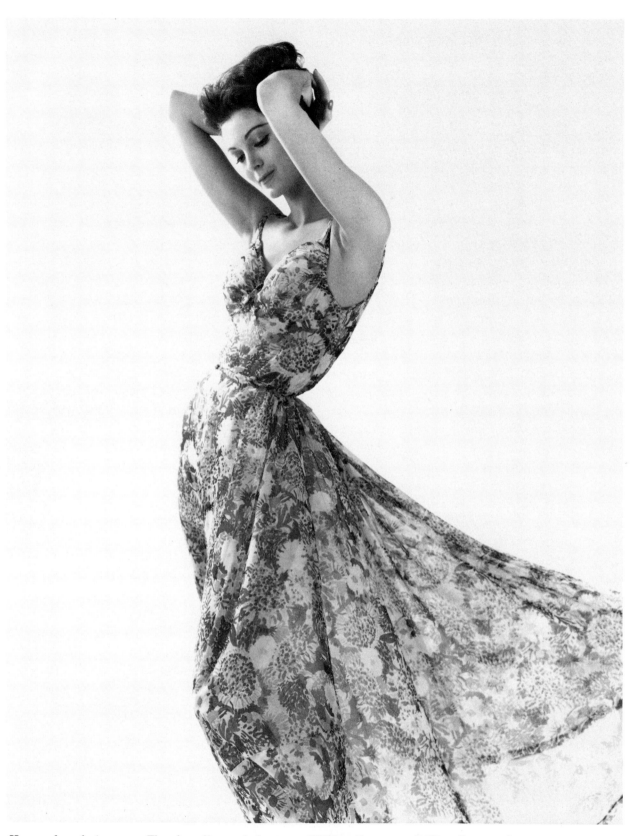

Here and on facing page: The clean line and elegance of Lillian Bassman. *(Lillian Bassman)*

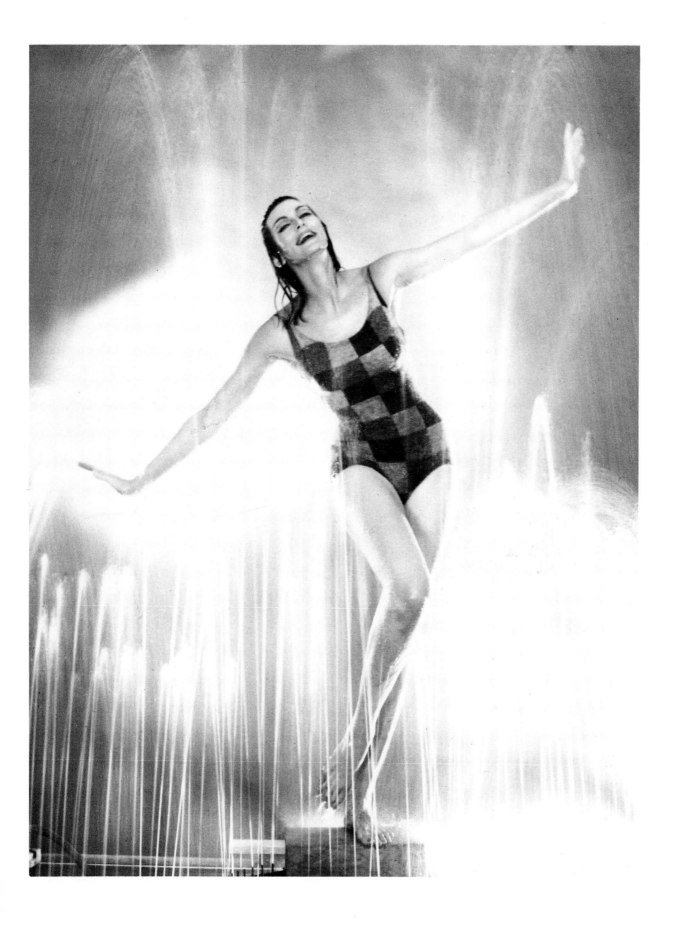

to *Harper's Bazaar* and another set of photographers with fresh points of view about me and what they wanted in their pictures. It was Derujinsky, Palumbo, Schiavone, Bassman, and Avedon. Of the lot, Lillian Bassman was my favorite, and most of the models who worked with her shared my feelings. She made us feel secure and important as individuals and not simply as objects in a photographic composition. Fluid simplicity, elegance, and a clean line devoid of gimmickry were her special qualities. We became friends, as did our children, and that friendship has endured. Lillian has enriched my life with a vision of the good thing that a loving and independent woman can make of the world around her without sacrifice of either career or marriage.

And now we come to Avedon. In my opinion, Richard Avedon is the greatest American fashion photographer of his generation. I had done a few advertising sittings for him in the past, but we had never really worked together. Not only were we under contract to different magazines, but I was not his type. I was too Latin-looking and too large in every dimension. When he finally sat me down and asked if I was ready to go with him, it was a thrilling moment. I suspect he did it because he had already gone through all of the other girls who had come up with me, and there was nobody else left of the old-school models with whom he did some of his best work. His motivation did not matter; like every model in the world, I longed to work with him.

It was spring 1957, and the first big Avedon job was to be on location in Paris shooting the new haute couture collection. I had done the collection the year before with another photographer, but I knew this was going to be different. We were both keyed up by the challenge of it. The previous Paris shoot had been professional, but nothing more. I wanted this one to be triumphant. I also wanted to prove that Avedon could use me every bit as effectively as he had my predecessors in the same locale, and the

list was formidable. It included every great modeling name of the day: Dovima, Dorian Leigh, Suzy Parker, Sunny Harnett, and many more.

For Avedon, finding a new way to see the city was the challenge. He had done so much work there, most memorably as adviser on the film *Funny Face*, the year before. It was a musical built around shooting the collection, with Fred Astaire playing a character not so loosely based on Dick Avedon.

Avedon taught me more about makeup than any cosmetician. He studied my face with a sculptor's eye, insisting that I thin out my eyebrows and go to an electrologist to have my hairline raised, a practice I kept up for years until the hair died and it was no longer necessary. By the time we left for Paris, he had re-created Carmen in accord with his image of her. It was an image I found eminently satisfying, and I stayed with it throughout this second high-fashion career.

That year the collection had a very romantic look, and the photographer unearthed a *belle époque* vision of Paris that was completely in tune with it. The photographs were not only among the best ever taken of me but were in my opinion among the best examples of Avedon's work of the period. He must agree, because they were prominently featured a few years ago in the large Metropolitan Museum of Art Avedon retrospective. The following year, a wall of photographs of me formed a part of the British National Portrait Gallery show of Parkinson's work. The fact that my image has played a role in some genuine examples of photographic art is the greatest reward my career has bestowed upon me.

Facing page and on the following three pages: The famous Richard Avedon Paris location for *Harper's Bazaar*. The picture on facing page adorned the wall of the Metropolitan Museum during the Avedon retrospective in 1982. *(Avedon)*

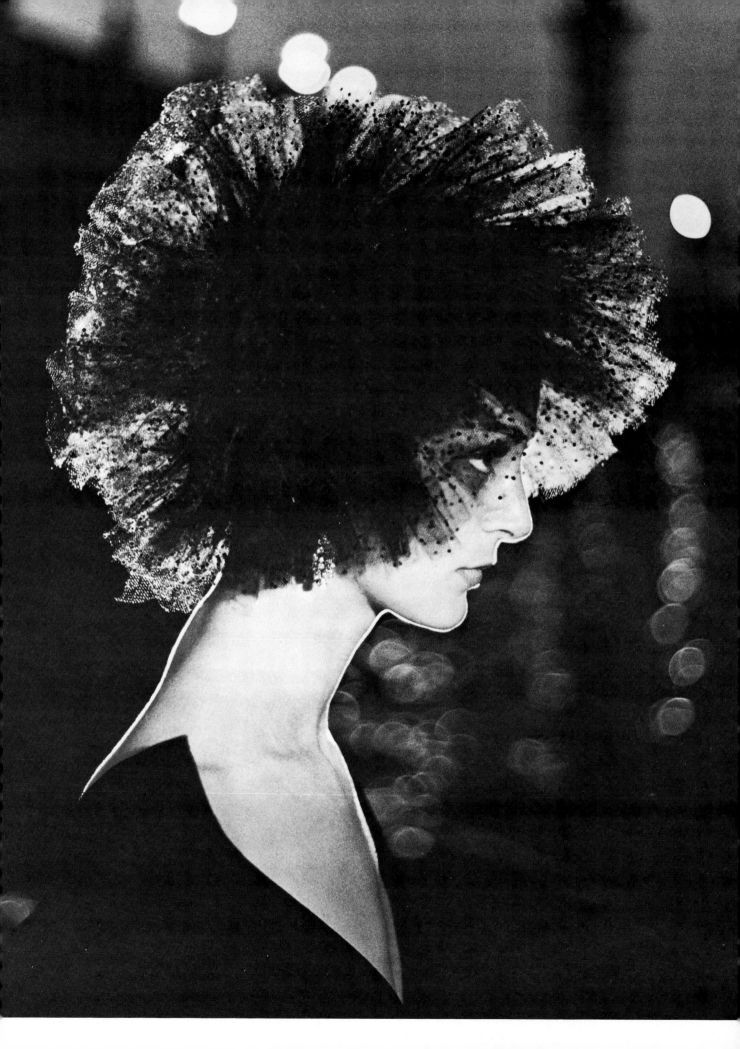

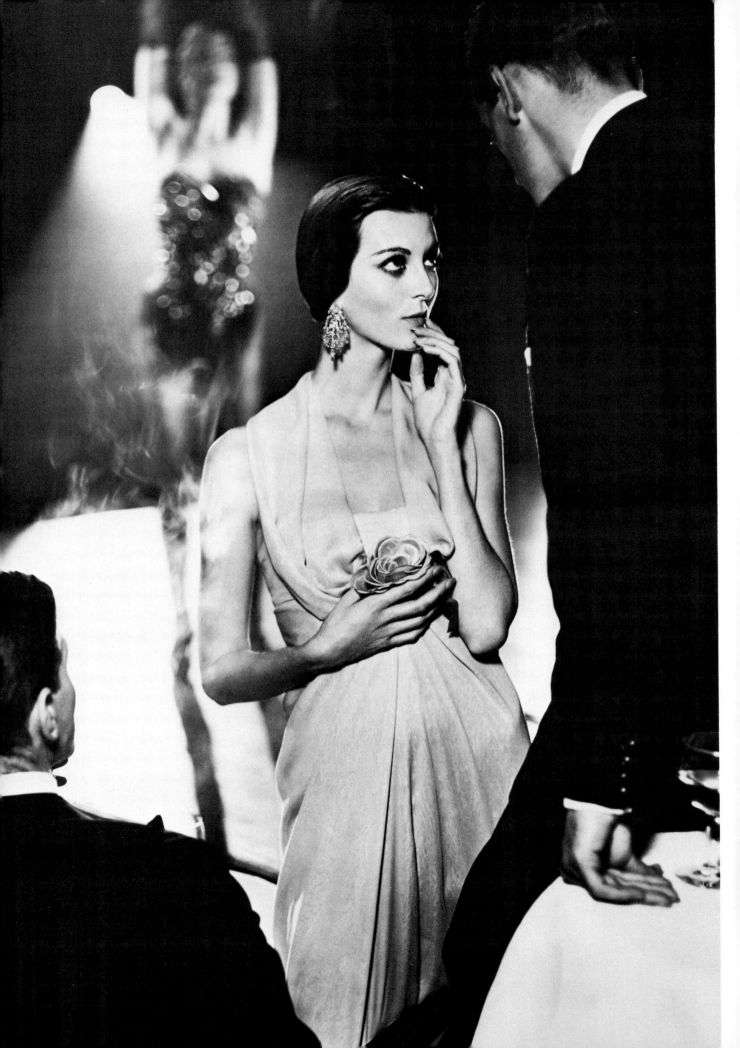

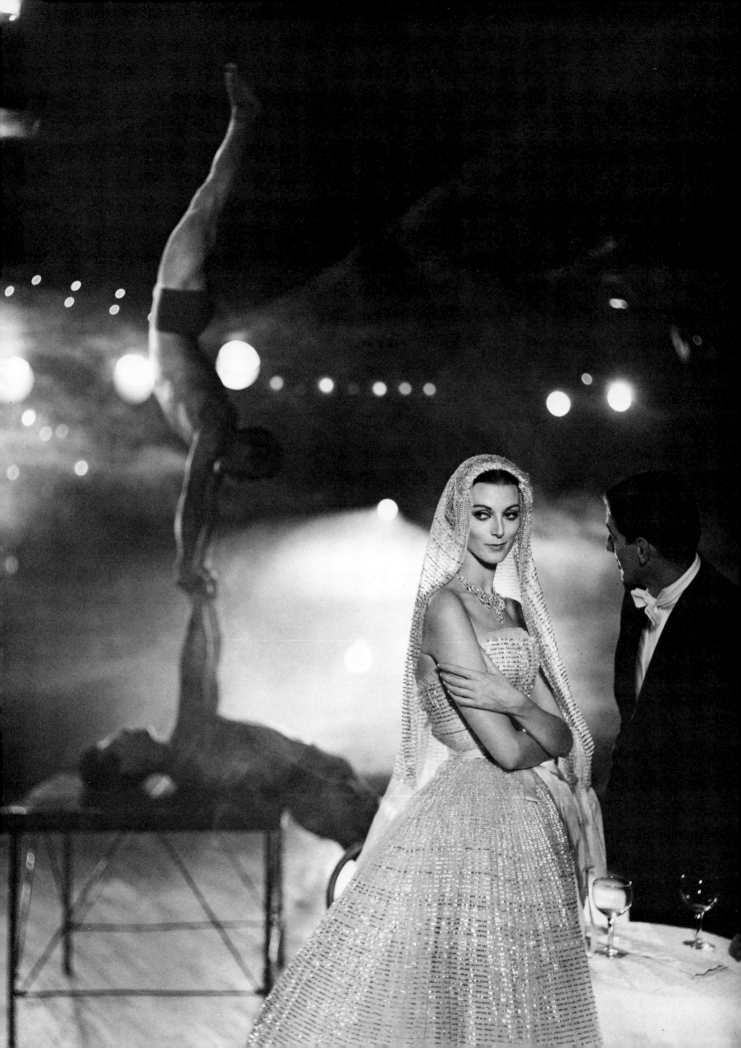

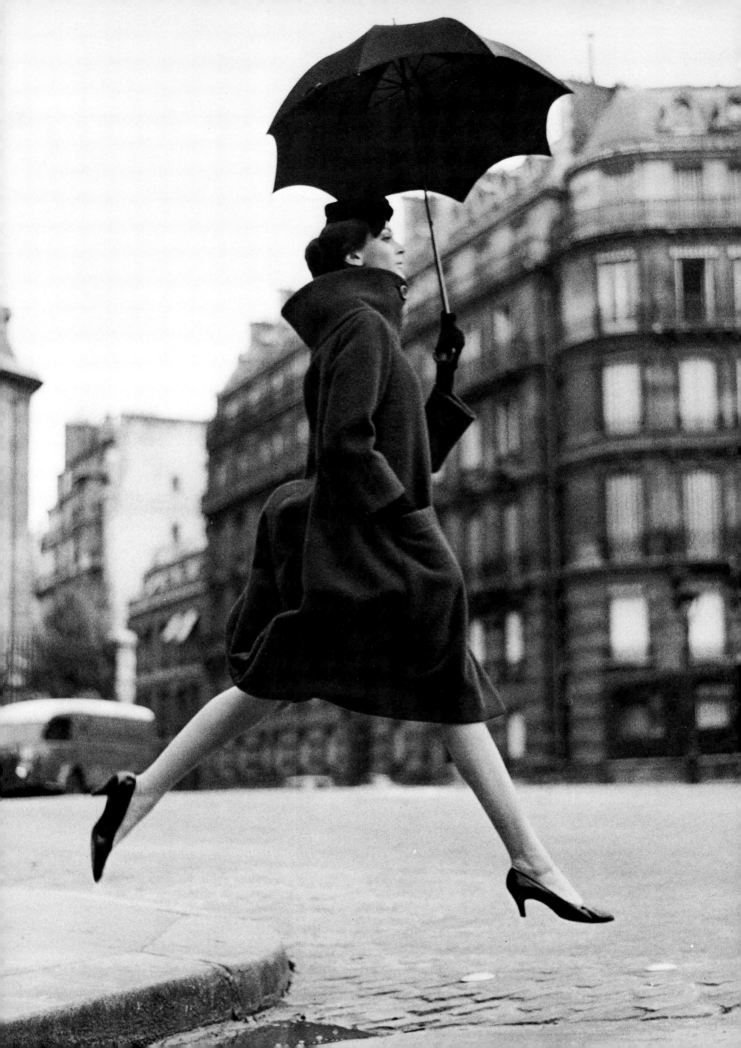

III

The first time I got married, it was to learn, and I chose an older man who was a natural teacher. Bill instructed me in all of the finer points of living well. He provided the opportunity and space that enabled me to develop my own taste and flair.

The second time I got married, it was for sex —basic fun and games with a man who seemed to be the perfect playmate. I'll never forget my first glimpse of Richard Heimann. He was shirtless, wearing only a pair of chino pants and the Rolleiflex hanging around his neck. There was this expanse of smooth, muscled, tan flesh, and when he looked up and flashed those expensive white caps at me, I was sixteen years old all over again. I had never seen such a gorgeous piece of masculine merchandise before. It was just too good to be true, and the first words I ever said to him were "Why do all the best-looking men have to be gay?"

He was just finishing a session with another model, and the beautiful blonde in front of the camera laughed convulsively. She was still laughing when she left the studio. Later, I learned she was his mistress and knew how wrong I was.

Had Eileen Ford not insisted, I probably would not have met Heimann, or at least not at the moment in our lives when we were both so ready for each other. It was a hot August day in 1958. I had just returned from a location shoot with Schiavone in still hotter Tahiti, and I was both tired and disgruntled. Eileen called to say she had a booking for me in what is now known as Chelsea. I was living at 16 East Ninety-sixth Street and told her it would have to be something very special to get me downtown that afternoon. "Cancel the booking," I said, then paused to think and added, "Unless, of course, it's Avedon."

She asked me to do the job as a favor to her. This was a new photographer and she wanted to help him get started. Eileen must have been as captivated by Heimann as I later was, for it was not the kind of thing she ordinarily did. I was one of her top clients and usually reserved for the best jobs with the leading photographers. My time was big money and not something she wasted on newcomers. When Eileen asked you to do something for her, you did it (at least, I did) because she rarely asked anything unreasonable.

It was not until after this first booking that I discovered how good Heimann was. At the time, I was conscious only of compelling green eyes, thick dark hair, and this incredible animal magnetism. I knew he was pulling out all the stops for me, but I also knew it was working.

In Heimann's eyes, I was a star, and he couldn't believe I actually had agreed to do the job. It was only an hour booking in an inexpensive, forgettable dress for a one-shot ad, but it was very important to him. After we finished, he took me down and put me in a cab, which I thought was a very nice touch. Most photographers barely grunt as you go out the door. He said, "Listen, can I call you for dinner sometime?" And I replied, "I thought you'd never ask." I took out the only piece of paper I had— a map of Tahiti—and wrote my number on it. That was late August, and we were married on February 15.

We got along on so many levels. He was wonderful with Laura and a sensitive, perceptive, creative person.

Alas, he was also twenty-six, a year and a half younger than I, which, as Dr. Kinsey reports, is very good for the sex life, but which, as I'm here to report, is not so good for the day-to-day living, especially when the woman is making much more money and is much better known by the people in the man's own profession.

As a photographer, Richard Heimann had a unique visual image of me. There was an under-

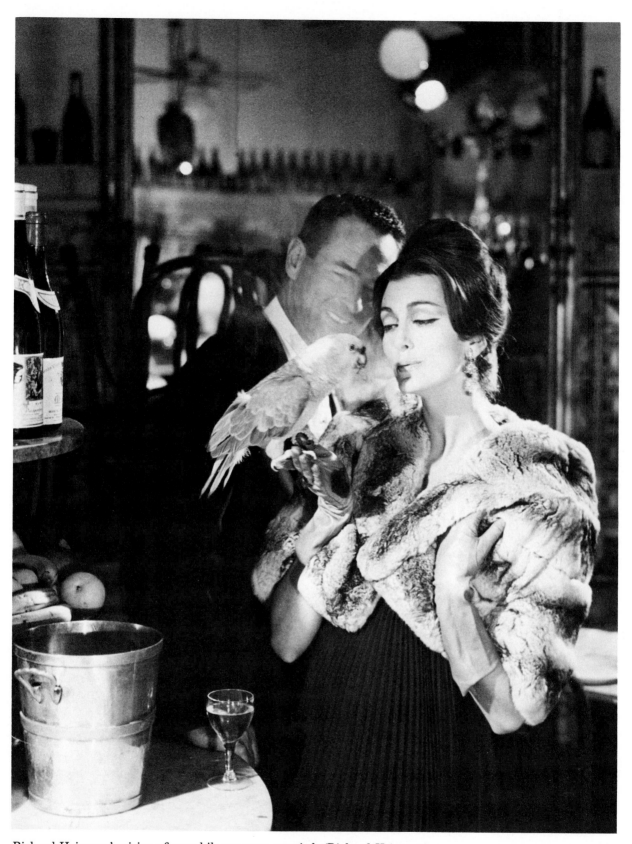

Richard Heimann's vision of me while we were married. *(Richard Heimann)*

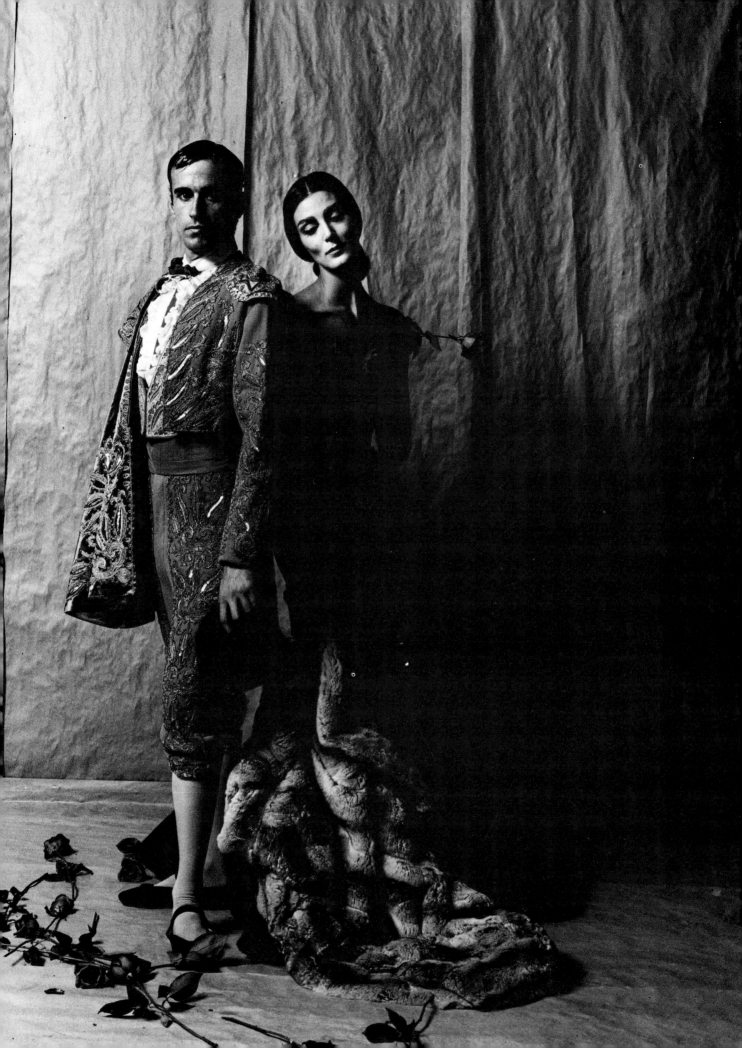

lay of eroticism in his pictures that no other photographer had captured. It was not an overt sexuality but an availability, a sensualness that occasionally bordered on a perverse sadomasochism. He knew what he was looking for in the lens, and he found it. He was a very good photographer with a particular visual point of view, which he achieved through an understanding of lighting and of the mechanical limitations of the camera.

When we got married, we were at opposite ends of our careers. I was at the top with fifteen years of success behind me, and he was just starting out. His business began to pick up rapidly when it became known that he could get Carmen for the job. We worked together a great deal, and at first it was fun. We would go on locations that were half shoot and half vacation. I'd put off other jobs because I preferred to work with him. We were having a very good time, but as his reputation grew and mine began to slip due to my unavailability to other photographers, a change started to take place. Working for him became increasingly difficult. There was a competitiveness that was close to aggression and often spilled over into rudeness. I didn't understand then what is so clear now: Richard knew how good the work he was turning in was; and the better it became, the more he seemed to resent the fact that often he got opportunities only because I was part of the package.

I decided to stay home more and leave the breadwinning to him. It wasn't an effort to save our marriage, because I didn't really feel it was in danger. I loved to cook, and decorate, and be there when Laura came home from school. But it was not what Richard wanted, and only made things worse. In a sense, a model is a photographer's fantasy, and when men marry their fantasies, the relationship disintegrates when the fantasy dissolves to reality.

Richard left. I had not expected that, had not expected to fail. Thinking he would return, that

56

all he wanted was a little space for himself, I put off telling Laura. She adored him, and I knew once I told her, it would really be the end; it would be too cruel to keep raising and lowering her expectations. But the time came when it could be put off no longer. The marriage was over.

I had to go back to work to support my child. I was thirty-two, a good age for most women but terrifying for a model, especially a model who had lost interest in her career because she had lost interest in herself. I was disoriented, had no plans, no order, no priorities beyond Laura's needs. Had it not been for my friends, both in the business and out of it, I would have been finished. They pulled me together and started me back to work. Things picked up, but never to the level they were at before Richard. The country was on the verge of a love affair with youth such as the world had never seen. At my age, I was lucky to be making a living in a business constantly searching for fresh and ever younger faces.

The emotional depression lingered. I was a member of a generation of women who still found their identities through men, and I had been devastatingly rejected by the one I loved. I wanted and needed to be loved, to be reassured of my worth in a man's eyes. Enter Richard Kaplan, smiling and swinging the proverbial tennis racket.

The second Richard was charming, witty, intelligent, a promising architect, and the son of a multimillionaire. More important, he thought I was the most beautiful girl in the world, and he was very much in love. Who could ask for anything more? At that moment, I certainly could not. We met on May 22, 1963; my divorce from Heimann came through in June; we were

Parkinson to the rescue when I had to go back to work after the breakup of my marriage to Heimann. *(Norman Parkinson)*

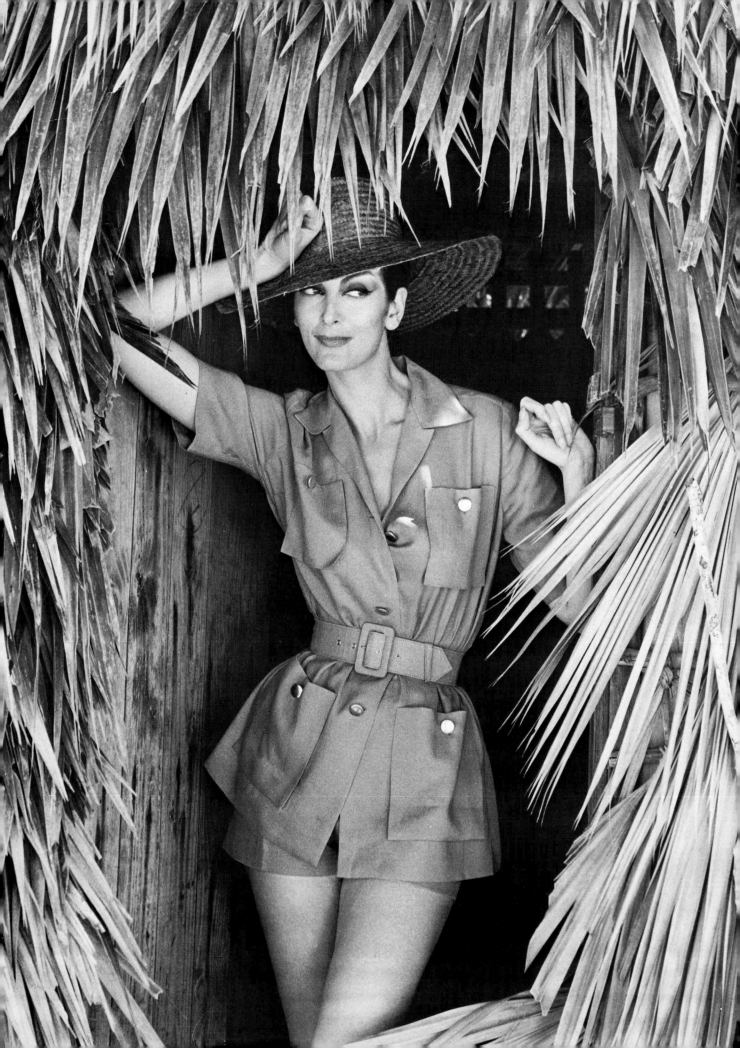

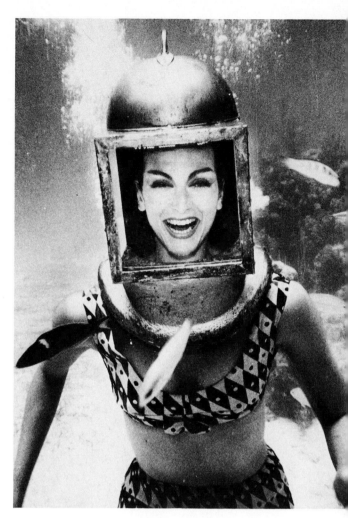

An underwater shoot with
Norman Parkinson. Parkinson is
the one with the moustache.
(*Norman Parkinson*)

married on October 6. I did not stop working.
Seeing my pictures in magazines pleased Richard II. It was as if it reassured him that he had
made the right choice. Although it seemed a
little childish, it was also endearing.

In 1964, we were about to leave for a vacation
in Greece when Paramount Pictures called and
asked if I could come to the Coast to play a part
in *The Last of the Secret Agents.* I had tested for
them in 1960, for *Breakfast at Tiffany's,* but had
not won the part because, at the time, they
thought I looked too much like the leading lady,
Audrey Hepburn. Apparently, however, the test
was good enough for them to take another look
at it four years later.

Richard offered to come to California with
me instead of going to Greece. He remarked
that, at my age, I might never get another opportunity, and if I didn't go, I would always
think he kept me from it. It was all said very
lightly—he was being funny, not nasty—but
there was this subtle undertone, a suggestion
that I might be over the hill. It lingered long
after the picture was completed and had failed
at the box office so dismally you don't even see
it on late-night television.

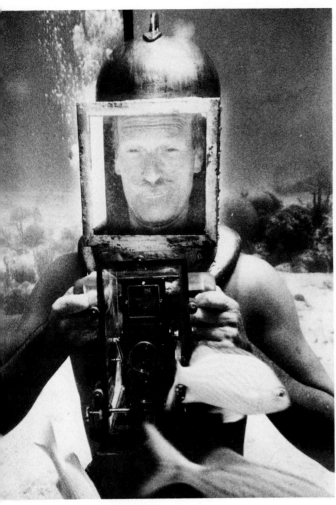
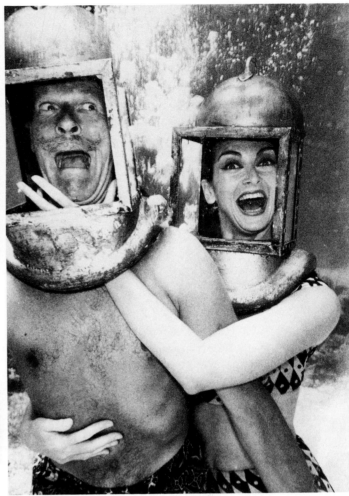

By 1966, whether Richard had meant it or not, I thought the implication was right. It was time to quit. I had already had the best of modeling. Twenty years of being on or near the top was a very good run, and most of my contemporaries were already out of the game. Eileen had some jobs lined up, and I called to tell her to book out. She asked how long I would be unavailable. I replied, "Forever."

The late Sixties was a period of complete upheaval, and it confused and frightened me. I did not understand what was happening and clung to the old-fashioned verities as if salvation and enlightenment could be found only in them. I stayed home and looked after my family. For diversion, I made a studio out of the maid's room in our triplex penthouse and began to paint again. We were building a house in the Hamptons and went there on weekends. Having both the ocean and a swimming pool was heaven. At thirty-five, I had become a middle-aged matron living a town-and-country life. It was bliss. My husband and I were so in tune, the rhythm of our life together like close harmony. It was, I thought, as it should be.

The world began to seep in so imperceptibly that at first I did not notice it. There was a small contretemps over the miniskirt, which was then all the rage. It was wrong for me—like most animals, I was best cut at the joint and not at midthigh—but Richard loved the new fashions and wanted to see me in them. It was too small an issue to fight over, and so I complied without ever feeling comfortable or liking the way I looked. It was so insignificant, it never occurred to me that it was symptomatic of worse to come.

Our friends seemed to be racing backward in age while at the same time shouting how modern and progressive they were. Drugs, promiscuity, rebellion against all of the old standards were the order of the day. It seemed ridiculous. I had not wanted to be as young as they longed to be even when I *was* that young. I thought Richard shared my opinion, but I was wrong. Youth had seduced him, and when he looked at me, he saw an older woman. He was not a deliberately cruel man, and nothing changed overnight. But change was coming.

I still have a photograph he took at about that time. In it, I'm not wearing a drop of makeup. I'm still bewildered when I look at it today. How could he have thought that face was too old for him? Yet he did. There were constant remarks on the natural changes that were taking place in my body. A pat on the bottom with the observation that it was dropping, not as firm as it used to be—always accompanied by a smile, a disarming and very boyish smile. I wondered if I was being hypersensitive, if I had been a "famous beauty" for so long that I couldn't take a little kidding about being somewhat less than I once was.

Then there was the incident of the hair. One morning, I rolled over in bed and Richard reached toward me. I thought he was going to embrace me, but instead his hand moved up to my head, and he plucked out a gray hair. He studied it with an expression of horror on his face. I had been getting gray since my early twenties and had lately been thinking the dyed dark hair was beginning to look hard on me. Gray is nature's way of softening at a time in a woman's life when her looks are enhanced by a softness around the face. I explained to Richard that I wanted to see how the natural gray would look. He replied that it would look old and awful. Get thee to the dye pots.

From bottom to head and finally to bosom. It was Richard's opinion that they were sagging. It was true my breasts were not what they were when I was nineteen, but he had not known me then and what he saw was no worse than they had been a few years earlier, when he was describing me as the most beautiful woman he had ever known. I had lost too much of my self-esteem to explain this adequately, and so I decided to visit a plastic surgeon for a bosom lift.

When I explained the situation, Dr. James MacDonald handled the matter with great tact and wisdom. He asked me to have photographs taken of my breasts and to bring my husband along on the next visit. Richard was embarrassed but agreed to return to the surgeon with me.

Dr. MacDonald explained the operational procedure and began to question Richard in a way that implied he thought there was nothing wrong with my body and could not understand why anybody would want me to tamper with it. When it was put to him in that way, my husband backed down, protesting he thought I was crazy to contemplate such surgery. Perhaps I *was* crazy: When you want to attack yourself physically just to please your husband, it is a form of desperation bordering on madness.

I was maturing in both face and figure. It was a natural change. The saddest part was that Richard could not recognize the compensating natural maturing that was taking place in my heart and mind. The marriage lingered on. I fought for it as hard as I knew how to fight, for, despite everything, I still loved him. It was a losing battle. What was happening in the streets

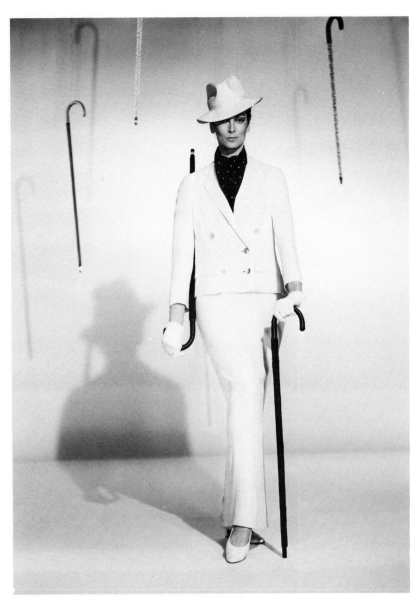

Publicity still for my movie, *The Last of the Secret Agents.* *(Paramount Pictures)*

had invaded our home, touching everything I held dear and turning it to ash. Richard had become much too young for me. There was nothing left, and we parted.

IV

If I had to choose the lowest point in my life, it would be 1973. My marriages had all been failures. I can now see that much of this was my own fault. It was a hangover from the modeling business. I was used to being subservient to a photographer's wishes, to being told what to do, to feeling only what they wanted me to feel. "Smile, Carmen." "Turn, Carmen." "Express romance, Carmen." "Give us some sex, Carmen." "Be a princess, Carmen." "Be a slut, Carmen." But it was never "Be Carmen," and so I never stopped to find out who she was.

I was forty-three. For the first time in my life, I was completely alone, without husband, or lover, or child, or parent. I had just enough

61

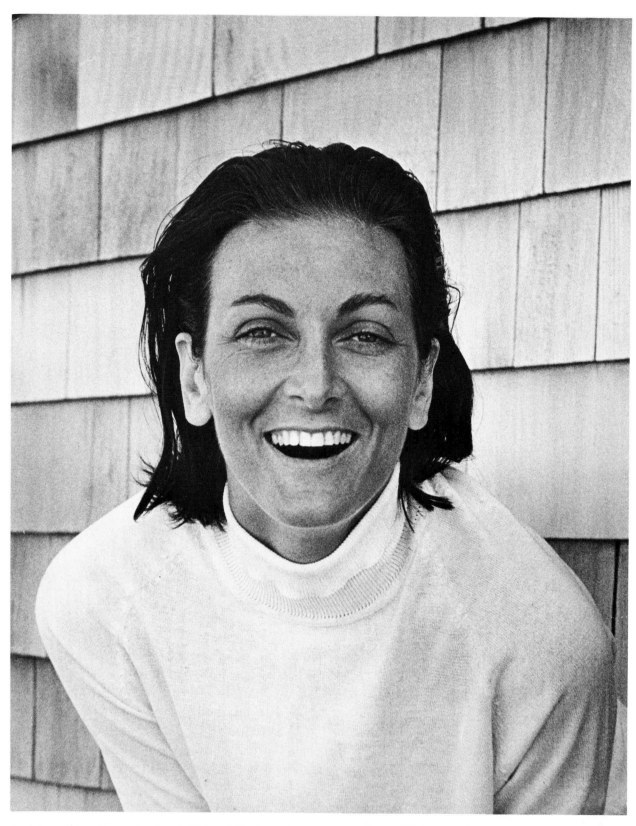

A picture taken by my husband, Richard Kaplan, at our summer home. Without makeup or hairdresser, you can see the start of those gray hairs. This is the unadorned face of the woman my 38-year-old husband was beginning to think looked too old for him.

money to get from day to day and no more. Perhaps I could become a booker at a model agency, one of those people who arranged time and jobs for models.

I made an appointment with Eileen Ford and dragged my fragmented self over to see her. She must have assumed I was trying to reactivate my modeling career, and before I could say a word, she clicked "Tsk, tsk, tsk," heaved a very heavy sigh, and said, "No, Carmen, no."

Ordinarily, a sense of humor might have asserted itself and I would have asked if she needed anybody to scrub the floors and empty the wastepaper baskets. There was no humor left, and I fled back to my shell. Eileen had only confirmed every doubt I had about myself, how little of value there was in me.

No woman walks away from three marital failures unscathed. No woman comes to what seems like the end of a brilliantly successful career without regret. No woman whose youth and beauty had brought fame and fortune terminates that period without fear. Those three climaxes were reached at the same moment in my forty-third year. I was scarred, rueful, and frightened. I became a windup doll operated by my friends. They took me in, fed me, found an apartment for me, tried to set me on my feet. I felt I couldn't move faster than I was going, which was standing still, so immobilized I couldn't even turn on a television set. It was as if something inside me thought I deserved what had happened to me. I had exploited my physiognomy without bothering to develop any inner resources, and now that stifled psyche had taken over and was punishing me. What had I succeeded at doing with my life beyond cashing in on a fortuitous accident of genetic structure? I felt humiliated, that I had nothing to offer that came from inside of me. I was only an image and an unwanted one at that. Oh, the maudlin glories of self-pity! It passes the time that has stopped moving.

Thank goodness, not everything was dead inside me. The survival instinct does not die easily and was slowly beginning to take over.

Without my knowing it, I was beginning to revive. I became aware of being cured upon awakening one morning to find that I was bored with the kindness and concern of loving friends. It seemed to have happened overnight, but of course it had been years.

It was time to do something, to take my life in my own hands. It suddenly occurred to me I'd never done that before; that it was not only five years of being adrift, I'd been floating along for all of my life. Even at the height of my career, I'd simply rolled with the currents, done what I was told, never resisted, never determined my own course. The time had come to battle the tides instead of letting them carry me where they would.

I examined my qualifications for various careers. Careers! That's a laugh—jobs: saleslady, secretary, receptionist, domestic engineer. No matter how I juggled the pluses and minuses, there was only one thing I was qualified for, one thing I had experience at, one thing I loved doing.

When I told people I wanted to go back to modeling, most of them looked at me as if my apathy had been replaced by total madness. Who the hell wanted a forty-seven-year-old model who didn't look like a grandmother? At sixteen I'd looked too old for *Seventeen* magazine, and at forty-seven I did not look old enough for *Modern Maturity.* The pervasive negativism had an opposite effect: It was exhilarating, a good-luck omen. New starts had always begun with predictions of doom.

I started networking in the business, and the first people who did not think I had taken leave of my senses were the photographers Schiavone and Hiro. They wanted to do some test shots. When Zoli, of the Zoli Modeling Agency, saw the pictures, his reaction was the exact opposite of Eileen Ford's. He said, "You look wonderful. I know there's a market out there for you. Let's find it."

Although it was a hard go at first, Zoli never gave up. The breakthrough was in 1980, when my darling Norman Parkinson came to my res-

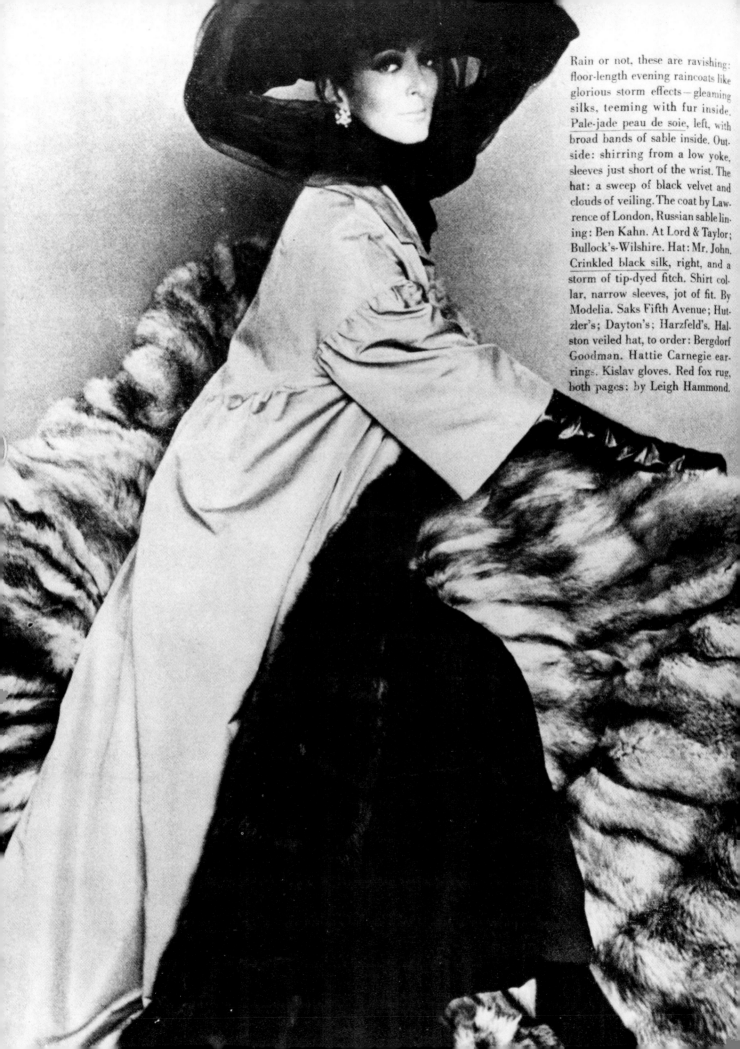

Rain or not, these are ravishing: floor-length evening raincoats like glorious storm effects—gleaming silks, teeming with fur inside. Pale-jade peau de soie, left, with broad bands of sable inside. Outside: shirring from a low yoke, sleeves just short of the wrist. The hat: a sweep of black velvet and clouds of veiling. The coat by Lawrence of London, Russian sable lining: Ben Kahn. At Lord & Taylor; Bullock's-Wilshire. Hat: Mr. John. Crinkled black silk, right, and a storm of tip-dyed fitch. Shirt collar, narrow sleeves, jot of fit. By Modelia. Saks Fifth Avenue; Hutzler's; Dayton's; Harzfeld's. Halston veiled hat, to order: Bergdorf Goodman. Hattie Carnegie earrings. Kislav gloves. Red fox rug, both pages: by Leigh Hammond.

cue like the knight on a white charger of my adolescent dreams. He told me to pack my bag and meet him in Paris. He was shooting the collections for French *Vogue.* It was the height of the magazine trend for using teen-age models in high fashion, but Parkinson was going to use quinquagenarian me.

When he got back to New York, Parkinson took the French *Vogue* pictures to Frank Zachary, the editor-in-chief of *Town & Country.* He handed them to Zachary and said, "Isn't it time for an elegant woman again?"

Zachary sent for me. He later told his Beauty, Health, and Special Projects editor, Nancy Tuck Gardiner, "Carmen is one of the very few models who aren't a disappointment in the flesh. She's just as beautiful in person as she is in her photographs."

Nancy is a beautiful young woman who has no hang-ups about gender or the generation gap. She has since opened many doors for me and gently nudged me through them.

One thinks of the fabled California estate San Simeon in terms of its creator, William Randolph Hearst, and *Town & Country* is one of the Hearst magazines. But the people in charge of the mansion had consistently refused to grant *Town & Country* or any other magazine permission to use San Simeon as a location for a fashion shoot. Zachary managed to persuade them to make an exception for Parkinson and me. We went off to California to create what was called "the Elegant Woman Portfolio."

San Simeon is Hearst's fantasy-come-true, a unique blend of the medieval and baroque, with a very special aura of power, romance, glamour, and mystery. It conjures up images of the golden age of Hollywood, with private train-loads of stars transported up the coast for weekend parties. There will never be another place like it, for there will never be another man with the special vision to create it.

Parkinson understood all that San Simeon symbolized, and he used me as a vehicle to capture its essence on film. To my way of thinking, the results were much more than a fashion layout and some of the greatest pictures ever taken of me; they were, quite simply, an evocation of the legend and mystery of San Simeon.

More than any other publication, *Town & Country* is responsible for the renaissance of my career. Frank Zachary and Nancy Tuck Gardiner keep dreaming up new locations for Parkinson and me. So far, they've also sent us on location to Newport and to the Bonaventure spa in Fort Lauderdale. Who knows what exciting assignment tomorrow may bring?

When I first thought of going back to work, I assumed I would be doing the older-woman number—the mother of the bride, the stylish senior—but as it turned out, I went right back to doing the high-fashion glamour things I'd been doing since my teens. I don't know how long it will last, but I have a good feeling about it. My experience has finally taught me that you have as many years at anything as you want to have, if you want it badly enough to go after it in a positive way.

Something else has happened to help me along the way. The world has finally realized that women over forty are not back numbers in terms of vitality, chic, and curiosity. It seems rather simpleminded of the fashion and beauty world to have taken so long to realize that the largest market for their wares are women of a certain age; women proud of their battle stripes, the maturity they have earned; women who will no longer be pressured into accepting the latest adolescent fashion craze.

Let's give a loud hurrah for the maturity that comes only with age. I have only one qualification about that: Maturity should never be confused with complaisance, an acceptance of the status quo. True maturity is the knowledge that there is always room for improvement and the time and ability to make it.

Living out an expensive fantasy in Helmut Newton's photograph taken for *Vogue.* (Helmut Newton)

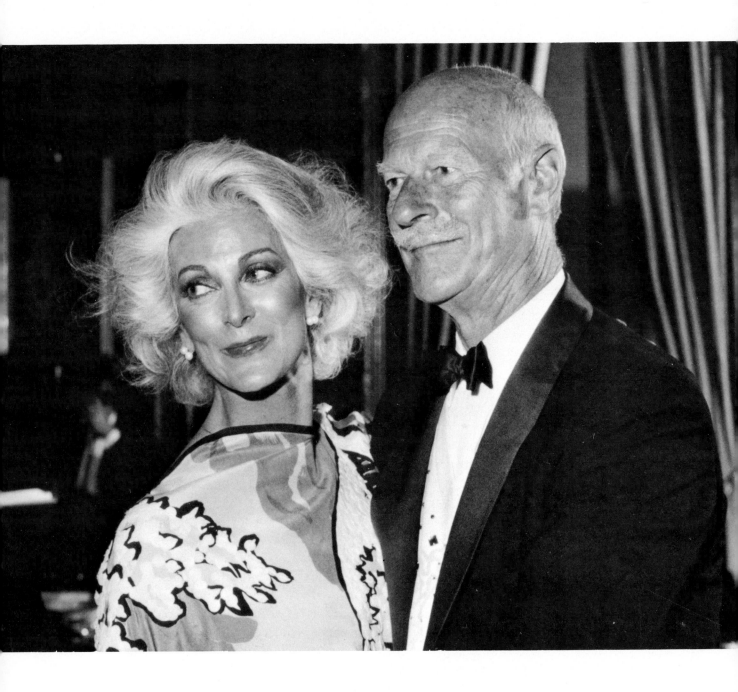

Parkinson leading the way—as usual. *(Bill Cunningham)*

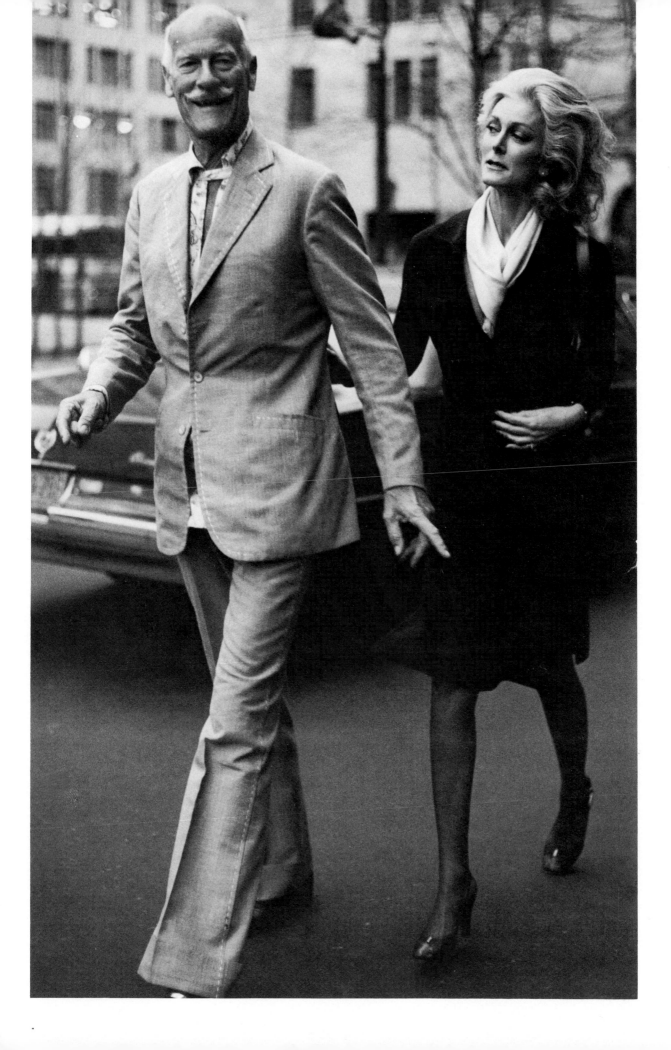

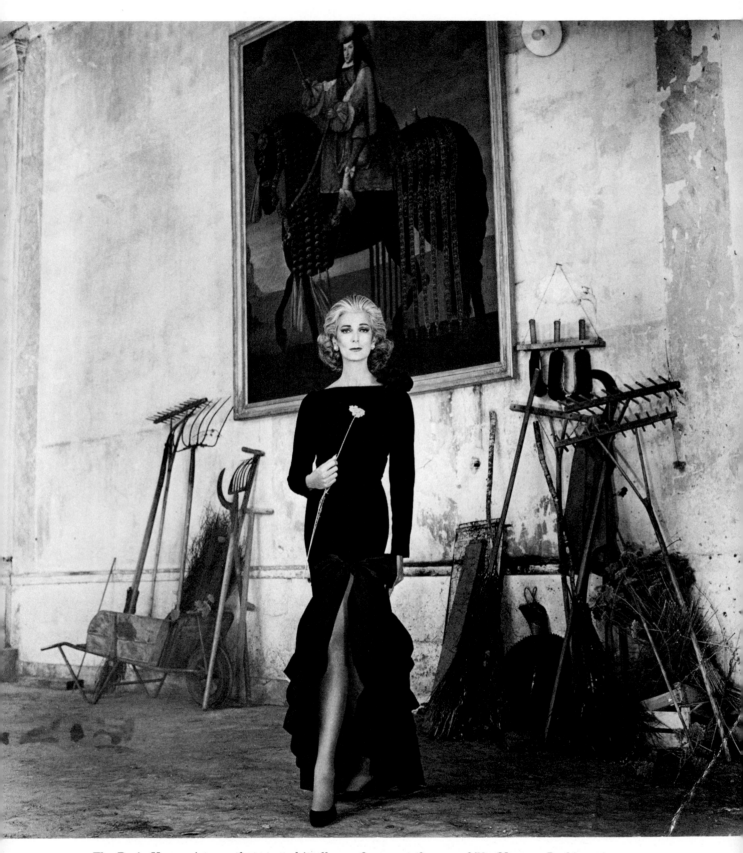

The Paris *Vogue* pictures that started it all over for me at the age of 50. *(Norman Parkinson)*

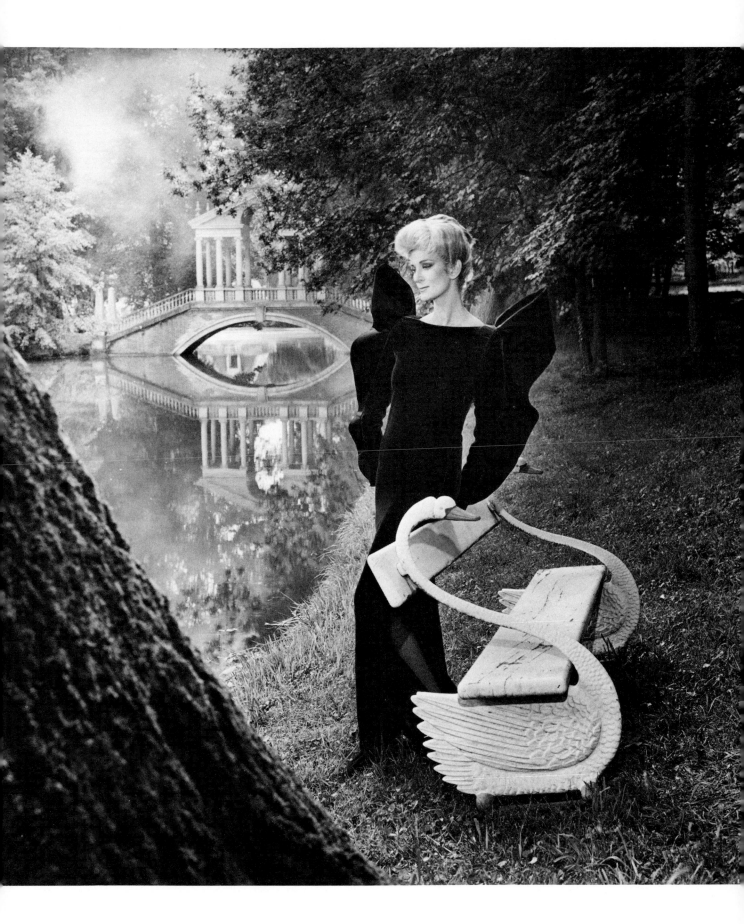

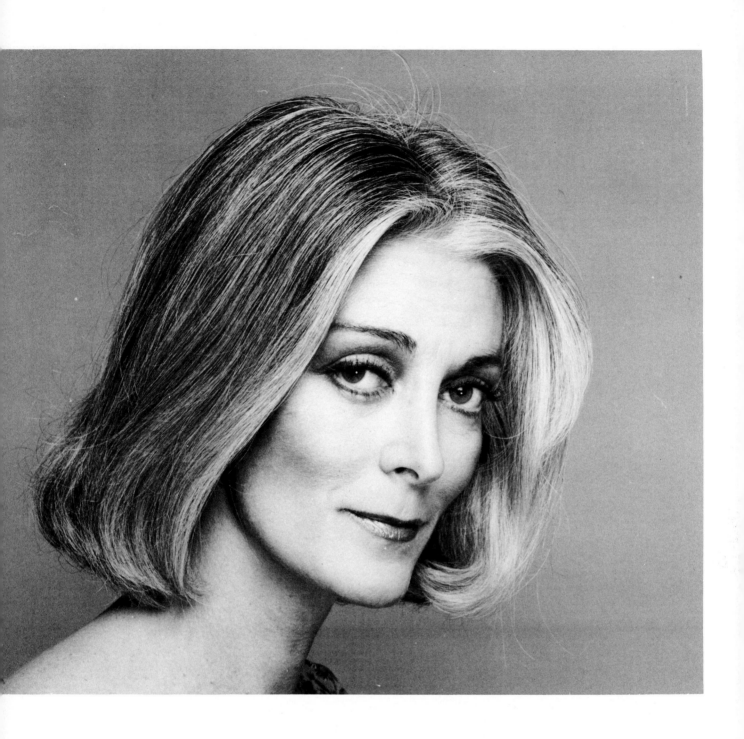

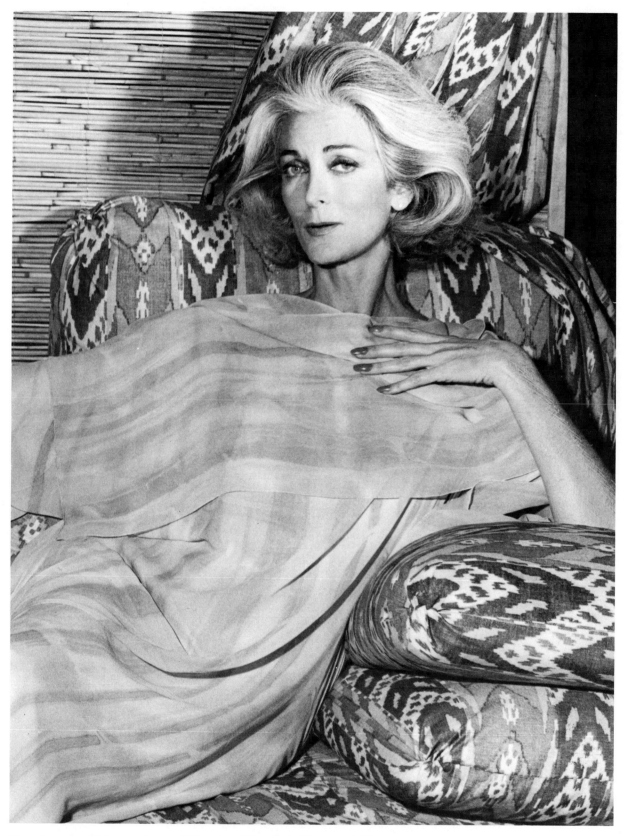

Test shots by Schiavone to see if I could still model. (Carmen Schiavone)

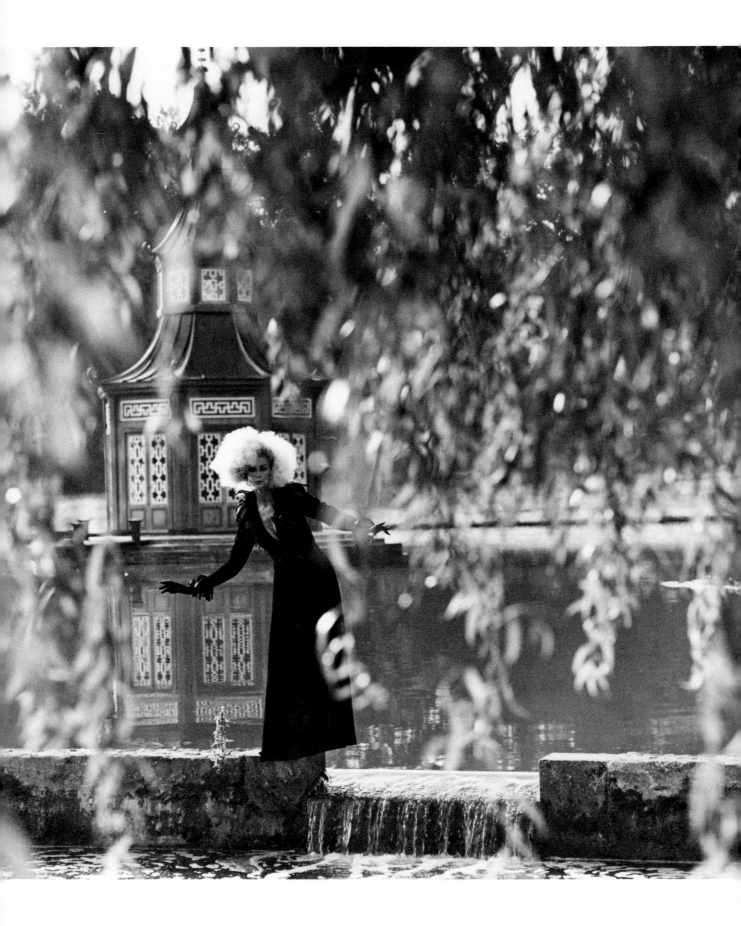

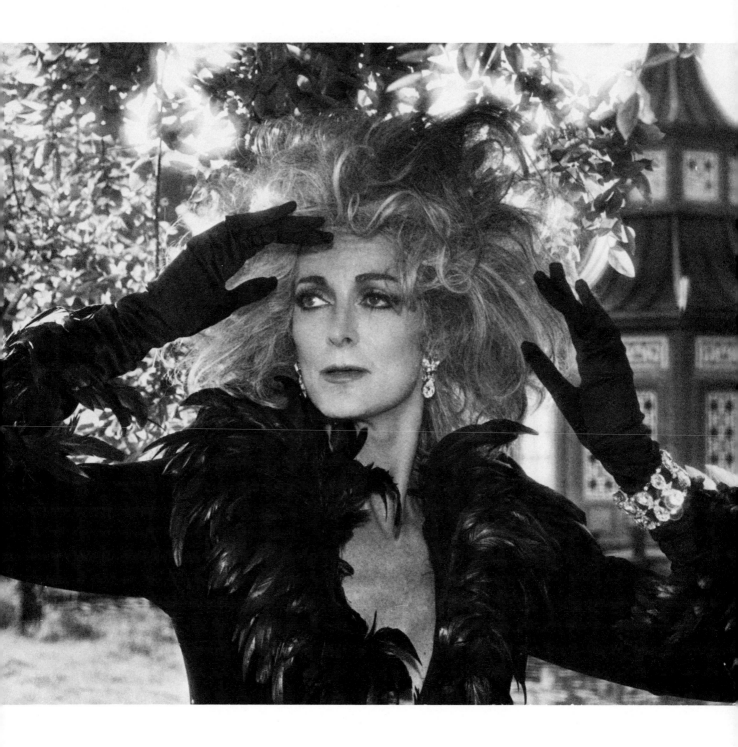

Two photographs in a series taken for French *Vogue* in
a villa outside Paris. (*Norman Parkinson*)

OVER 40
BEAUTIFUL BODY GUIDE

On these six pages, starting here with top model Carmen, all you need to know to take off years, pounds, inches with an ingenious diet and the ultimate body-shaping of dance. Plus, how four of the world's best dancers (all 40-plus) keep fit.

INSTANT FLAB-AWAY DIET

Thousands of women have dieted relentlessly, achieved their weight goal, but remained with areas of unsightly fat. Now, a new eating plan promises fast—and visible—results. That stubborn flab has a name—cellulite—and *Anushka's Complete Body Makeover Book* shows how to slim down and shape up permanently, as if you had actually attended one of the famous Anushka spas.

Authors Celestina Wallis and Ana Blau founded the first Anushka Health and Beauty Clinic in New York (the second is in Houston) to focus on the key trouble spots that are resistant to normal weight loss. The Clinics' name is derived from an endearing sobriquet for "Ana." According to Anushka's experts, cellulite—a disorder which afflicts only women—begins when tissues retain water, fats and wastes like a sponge. Once the process begins, it can be chronic and hard to reverse. Cellulite tends to accumulate in the hips, stomach, buttocks, thighs and sometimes the ankles, often impairing circulation.

The external signs: Skin appears pitted and bumpy, something like an orange rind, is usually dry and lacking in tone. Certain areas of the body appear out of proportion to total weight, most often leading to the "pear"-shape look women dread most.

WHAT CAN BE DONE?

Plenty. To dissolve cellulite deposits the specialists at Anushka have developed a personalized (CONTINUED ON PAGE 370)

Harper's Bazaar's September 1981 issue dedicated itself to the over-40 woman, highlighting a new, and growing, self-assurance among older women. *(James Moore)*

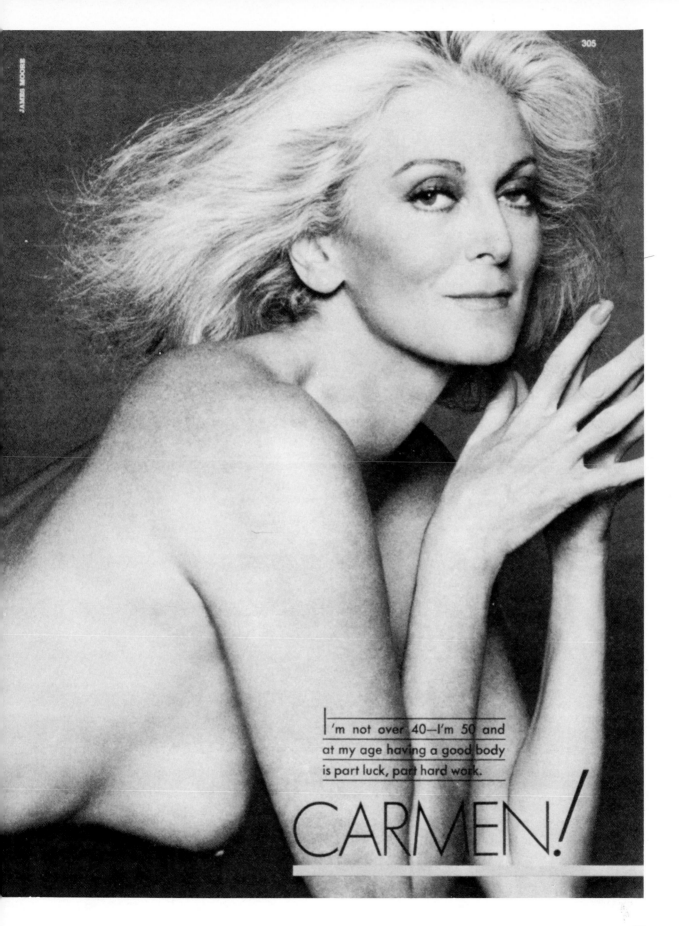

I'm not over 40—I'm 50 and at my age having a good body is part luck, part hard work.

CARMEN!

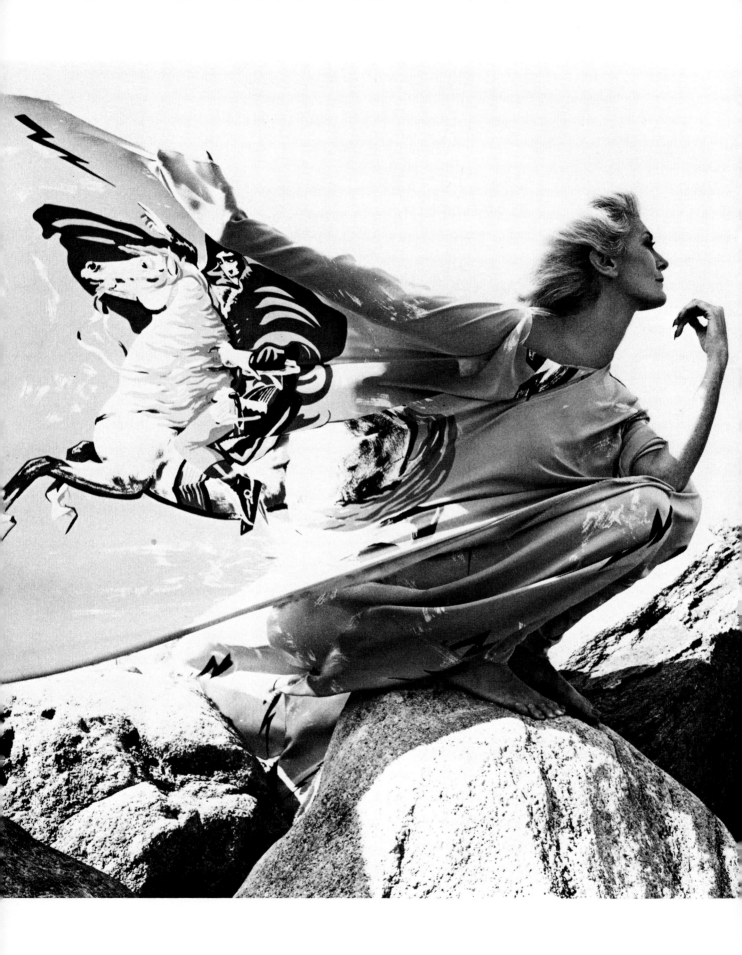

2

STARTING OVER

$\mathcal{A}$T FORTY-SEVEN, IT was difficult to decide to go back to modeling, but once the decision was made, a painful chore remained before it could be put into action. It was a question of taking stock. If modeling was the business, I was the inventory and the product. I had to see if I could compete with the newer and more streamlined models. That called for an objective appraisal of the pros and cons of face and figure. It turned out to be one of the most positive and useful things I've ever done, something I hope I would have done eventually even if I hadn't been contemplating a return to my career. It is the first piece of advice to any woman who wants to look her best.

All changes we want to be permanent and beneficial have to start on the inside and work

out to the surface. We may greet the world with the way we look, but we live with the way we feel.

Changes begin with the decision to change, and that can come only from the innermost part of you. They will not be lasting if they are only made because somebody else says we've gained weight, or are wearing the wrong makeup or clothes or what have you. That leads to a fleeting change which we probably make with a grudging "We hope our critics are satisfied" attitude. For changes to last, it has to be ourselves we please, an answer to self-criticism and personal evaluation.

The decision is made. It is a genuine cry from the heart. The next step is to try to rid ourselves of all the guilts and emotional garbage we women carry around along with our lipsticks and loose change. Let's get "they" out of our lives forever—the "they" who are wearing such and such this season, or doing, or saying, or

---

Perched phoenix-like on a rock in a Michael Vollbracht gown. *(Richard Corman)*

going. "They" are the good intentions with which the roads to our personal hells can be paved. Let's stop going that route. *I* wanted to look and feel better, and it had nothing to do with "they." "They" may have thought I was out of it, a back number, but let me tell you, after years of having to fall into step with the brass band of fashion, it was delicious to be marching to my own drummer.

Now that we've dealt with the decision and the arbiters, what do we do about the opinions of those we want to keep happy, and in our lives, but whose ideas on how we should look are somewhat questionable? I've told you about my third husband. He wanted me to look like a teeny-bopper, and I did try, just to please him. But it made me feel very insecure about myself, and the less secure I was, the less secure I became in our relationship.

There was another man who was very meaningful to me for a long time. He longed for me to look like the sexpot of the Western world and was happiest when his friends groaned with frustrated desire every time I was on the scene. I was not interested in anybody but him, but our affair came to an end very soon after I realized that he was more concerned about their envy of his good luck than about my desire to be attractive only to him. Through all the years of trying to please family, friends, and lovers, I've learned one lesson the hard way, and I'd like to pass it along: If someone really loves you, he will want you to be happy with *yourself,* as well as with him.

The happiest woman I've ever known is one who was so secure in who she was that she gambled on waiting for a man who did not want to change her in any way. Elaine had a beautiful face but was more than pleasingly plump; she was the definition of *zaftig.* Her mother and all of us who liked her were constantly after her to lose weight, but she was content with the way she looked and felt. She dismissed all criticism by saying there was one man in a thousand who liked a heavy woman; she would wait until he came along. He did, and they've been married for twenty-five years and raised three marvelous children. They are still completely in love. She remains a radiantly beautiful woman both inside and out because she has no problems with who she is or how she looks. Her style is stout, and she is the most stylish stout in town. To her husband, she is truly a great big beautiful doll.

We are all born wonderful individuals. Change begins with a recognition of who you are and what you want to do to improve that person. The most disastrous thing is to worry about whom you want to be, for you already are somebody. Trying to be somebody else is such a self-defeating waste of time. Save your energy for concentrating on *what* you want to be: slimmer, happier, stronger, healthier, more fulfilled in every area of your life. We are all individuals, and we should try to develop that individuality and not exhaust ourselves attempting to be somebody else.

Cherish what is fundamentally you and never be deluded by fashion's image of what you should be. Love who you really are. The essential you can be far more beautiful than any face in a magazine or on a screen. Don't try to assume the image of a movie star, or model, or socialite, or friend. You have your own image. It may have gotten tarnished and need some buffing and polishing, but it is there. Find it, recognize it, be happy with it.

I am the proof of what I am saying, for it happened to me. During those five years in which I lost the resilience that would have enabled me to overcome my emotional problems, the inner sag showed in every part of me. My hair lost its luster, my skin and body their firmness.

The first big practical step is to make friends with the mirror. It is counterproductive to look in it and be unhappy; what I saw was no longer what I had seen twenty years earlier. We have

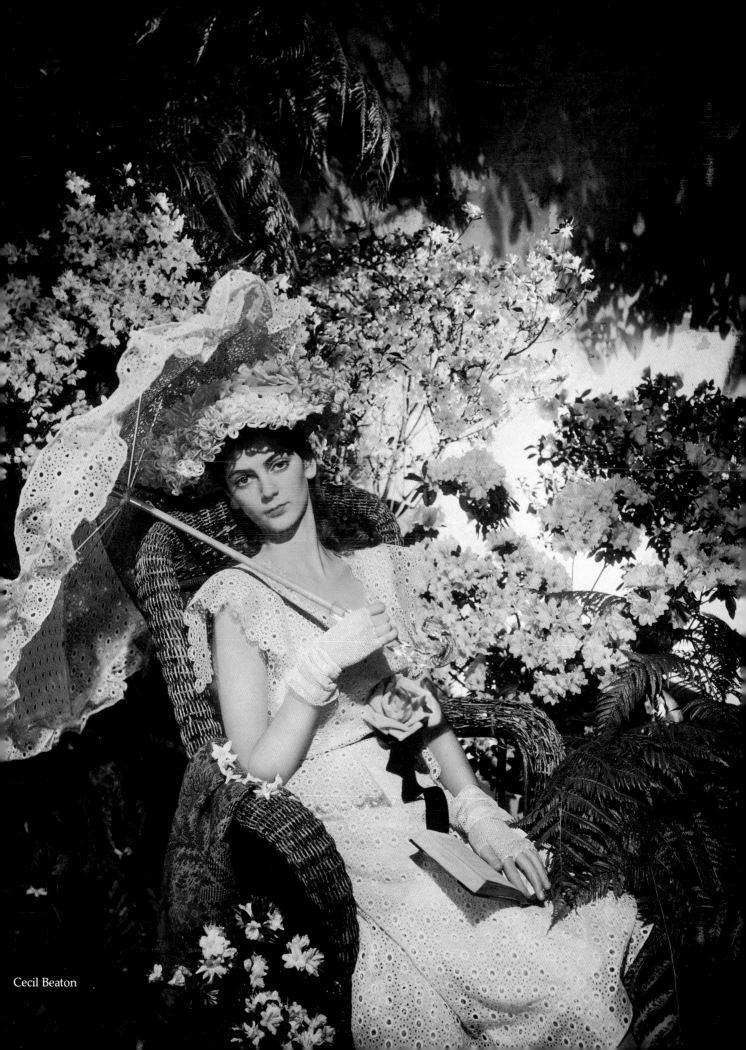

Cecil Beaton

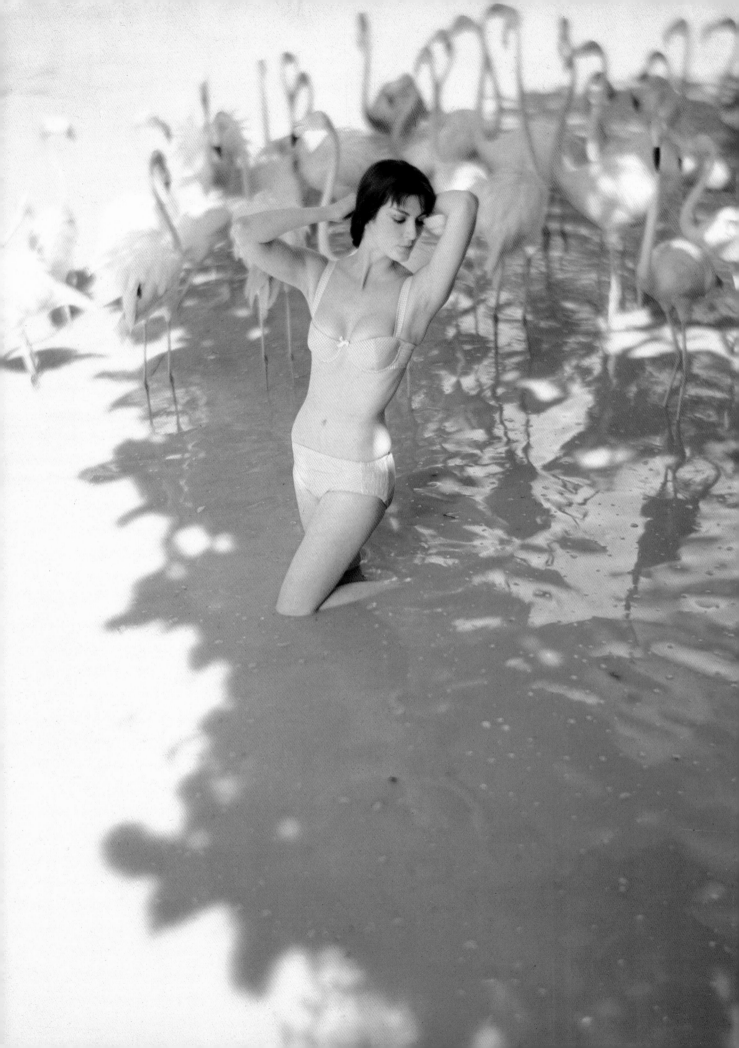

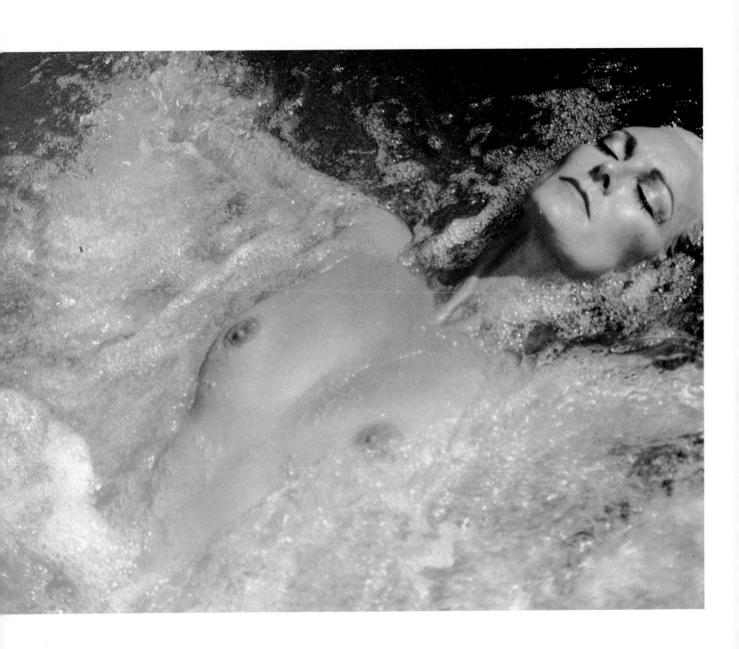

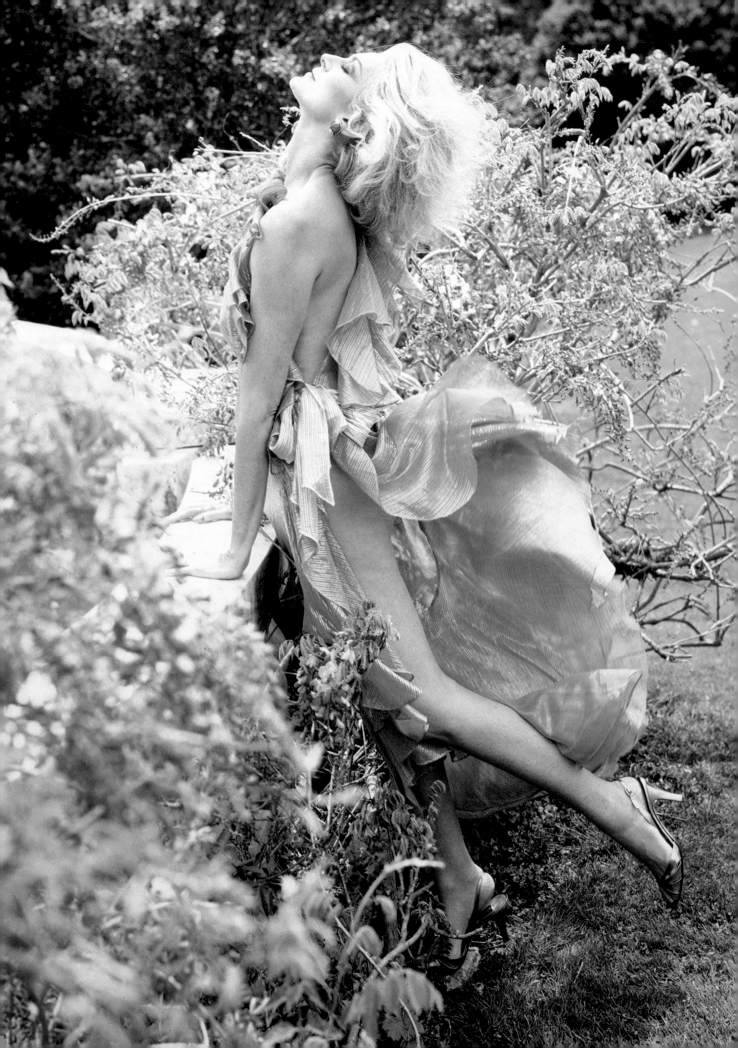

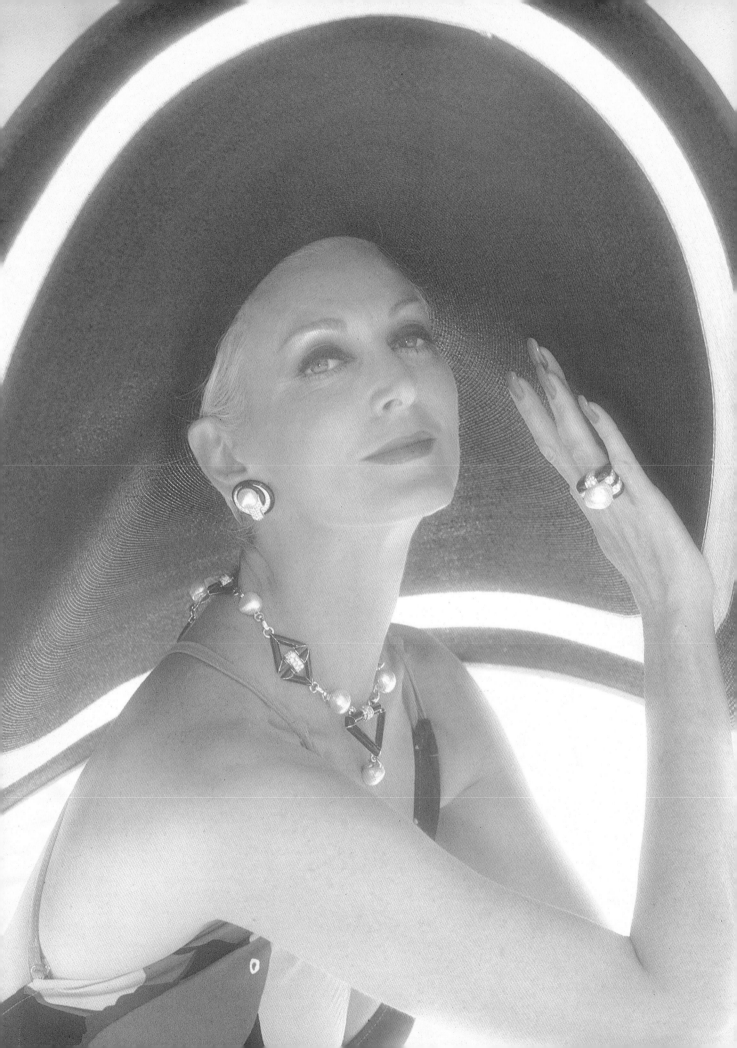

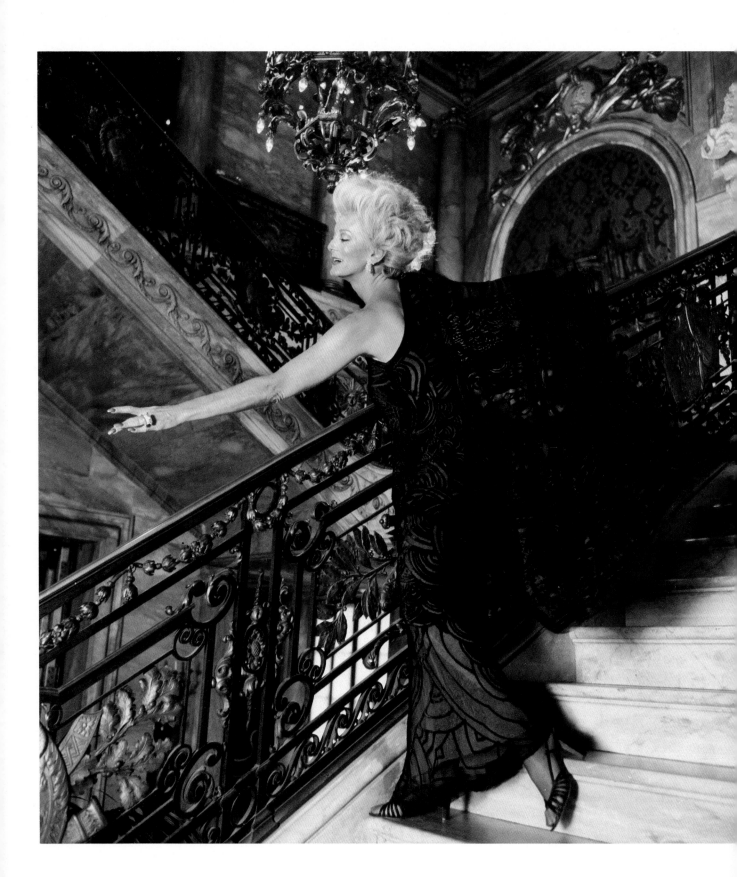

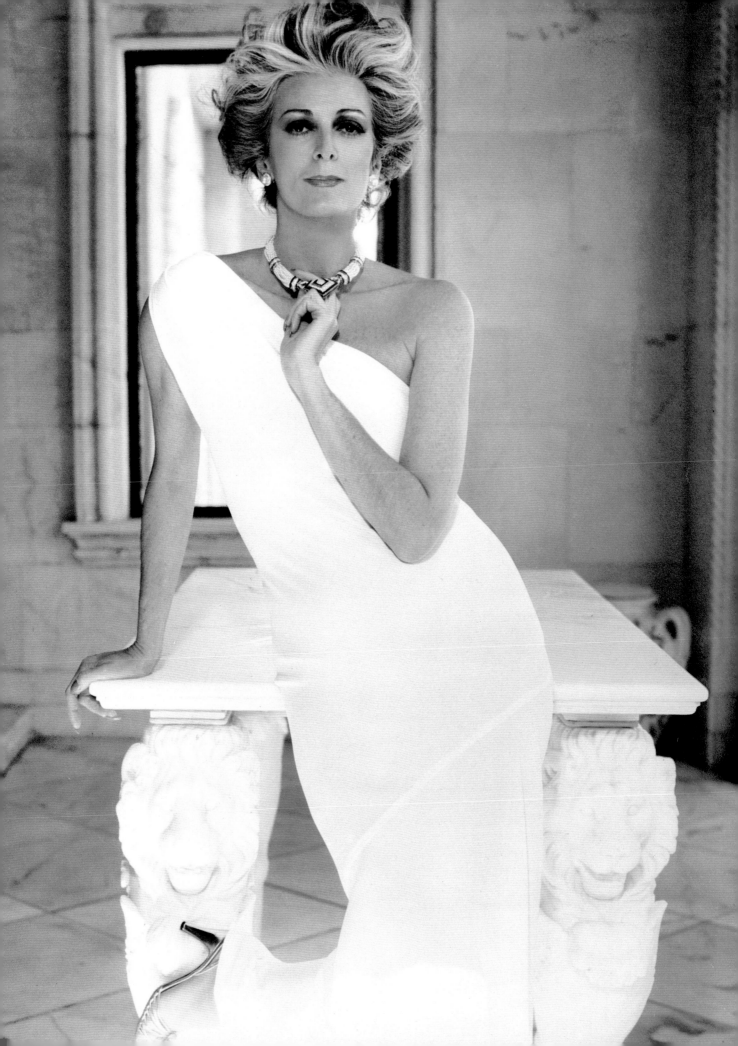

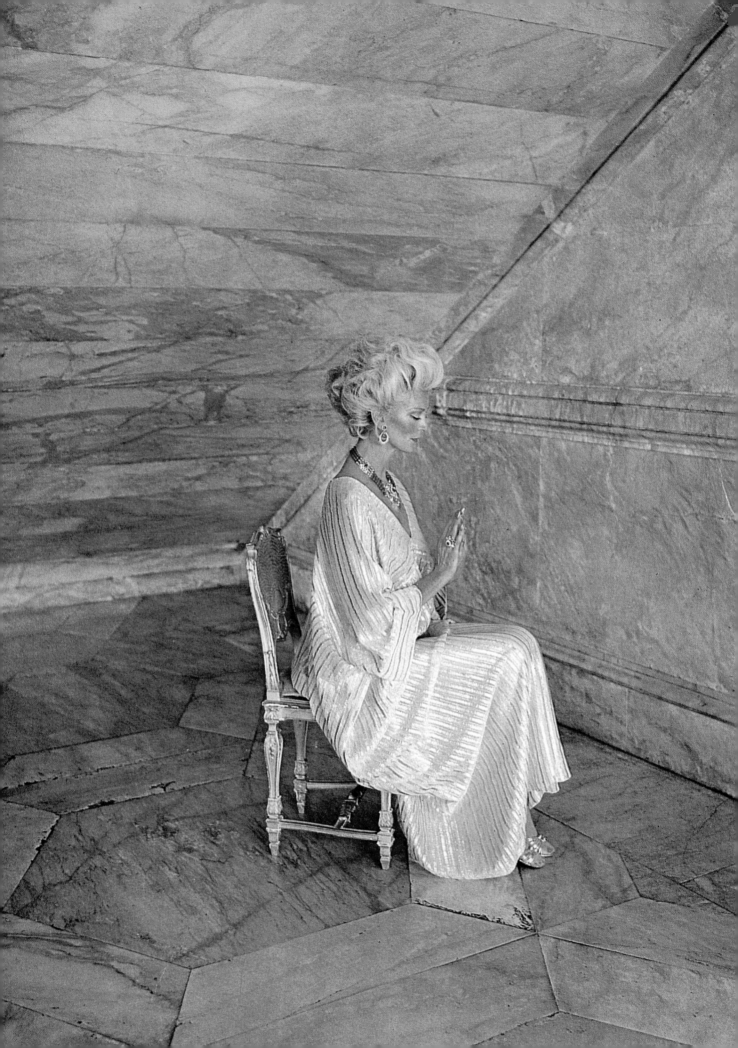

to stop being bullies and picking on ourselves for what is beyond retrieve; without a positive attitude, we cannot improve those things that make us unhappy. Be proud of all you've been through, and that includes the pains as well as the pleasures.

Look in that mirror and start with the positive. What am I happy with, and how can I make that still better? Improve your assets until you have enough emotional capital to cope with your liabilities.

In taking stock, a checklist of assets and liabilities is essential. What are immediately eliminated are the things that cannot be changed.

Most of us look in a single mirror. We concentrate on how we look as we enter a room or approach somebody. I studied my contemporaries and found they gave the greatest emphasis to their front and naturally best side. I recalled the importance of the mirrored studio in my ballet days. It was essential that we dancers see ourselves from every vantage point. We had to look graceful and assured from the rear and side as well as from the front.

My first and just about my only expenditure in starting over on a new regimen was to purchase a three-way mirror. If you have limited space, get one that folds away, or you can do what I did. I lined a wall of closets and shelves with mirrors that were actually three doors hinged so they moved in to become my three-way mirror. What I discovered on my first view of the total picture more than compensated for the not too great outlay of cash. It sent me scurrying back to my list of liabilities.

There was a roll of fat that I never knew existed, and there were sags just about everywhere. From the front, clothes and makeup made me look as good as I was capable of looking. From any other angle, I was much less attractive than I had to be. Clothes that I thought flattering hung in the most disfiguring ways. Oh, I know we all look in a three-way mirror in a dress salon, but what we're actually looking for most of the time are wrinkles in the dress, and how the hem hangs, and the fit of the sleeves. What my home investigation revealed were the wrinkles in me, the thickening in my upper arms, the trace of flab behind my knees. It was enlightening if discouraging. These were not irremediable flaws; it was simply that my old exercise routine did not extend to them, because they were not the problems of my twenty-year-old self. They would be prominent targets in the new one.

Set small goals, and don't expect overnight miracles. We have all the time we need, if we'll only stop wasting it by worrying about our age. Age is an inner thing. I measure my life by degrees of happiness and not the number of years I've been around. When I'm unhappy, I feel older than time; but when I'm happy, I have a fond but foolish feeling of immortality.

As I've said, I continued a beauty and exercise program through all of the years of my emotional paralysis. What I later discovered was that it was the wrong program. It was the one I had been using ever since Avedon helped to change my look. That was twenty years earlier, and the program was thus no longer valid. I had to start from scratch and find a program that would enhance the woman I had become rather than one that attempted to maintain me as the woman I no longer was. I was overdoing everything. The exercises were too strenuous, the skin care too abrasive, the makeup too harsh. All of this exertion was breaking down what was still good instead of improving it. I no longer had the energy, the physical features, and the mental outlook of my younger self. I had reached the balance of years, middle age, and had to find a balanced regime to harmonize with the contemporary me.

Fortunately, my career had provided access to an almost limitless amount of information on physical care. I did not discard all of my old, tried-and-true methods, but I did modify them,

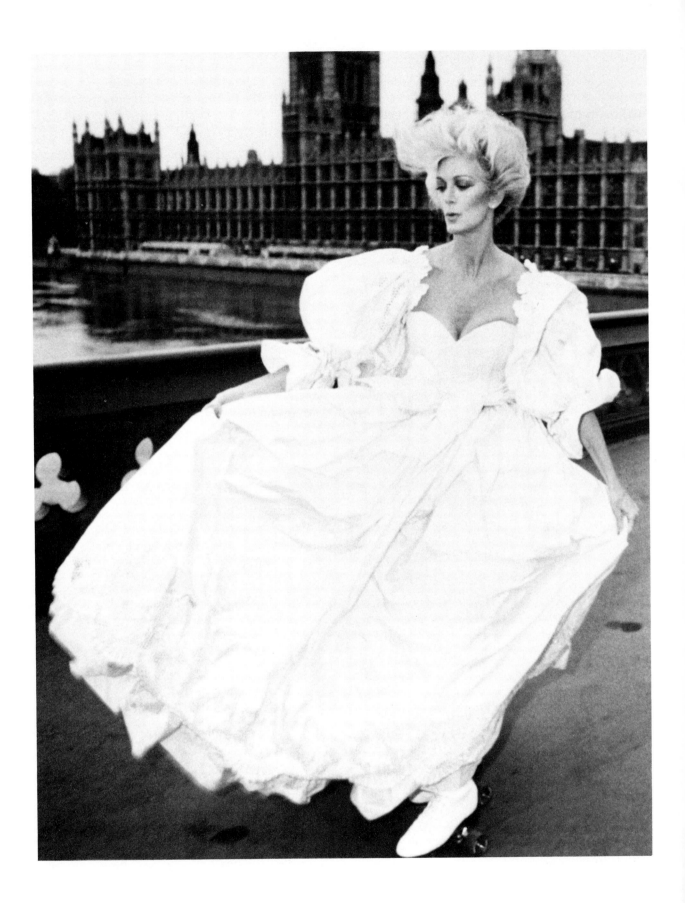

experimenting with new techniques and exercises until I came up with a synthesis that would work for any woman of my age. The result was a system of conditioning and treatment based on the golden mean. Drudgery was out. Less was always more in exercise, cosmetics, and diet.

We are now ready to get down to some specifics. Not everything I say will be right for you, nor should it be, for it would mean you had no assets, and I don't believe that's true of any woman. If our liabilities far exceed our assets, we are not counting properly. Let's go back and have another look and another thought about all of our sterling qualities. It is just as false to demean ourselves as it is to think we are flawless. None of us is without faults, but most of us are far better than we suspect.

This book contains something for everybody. How much and what that is depends on the reader. I do not believe in radical change but in gradual evolution, so leisurely that it becomes a part of us on every level of our existence. We did not get to our time in life overnight. We did not develop bad habits overnight. How foolish it would be to expect to change overnight. How doomed to failure is the crash diet or the crash anything else. Just think of the meaning of *crash:* to break into pieces violently and noisily; to shatter. Is that what you want a beauty regimen to do to you? Do you know anybody who walks away from a crash better off for the experience? What I want to give you is a slow and pleasant drive toward a destination you will be happy to reach.

Still roller-skating—this time across Westminster Bridge in London, in a ball gown by Princess Diana's favorite designers, the Emanuels. *(Norman Parkinson)*

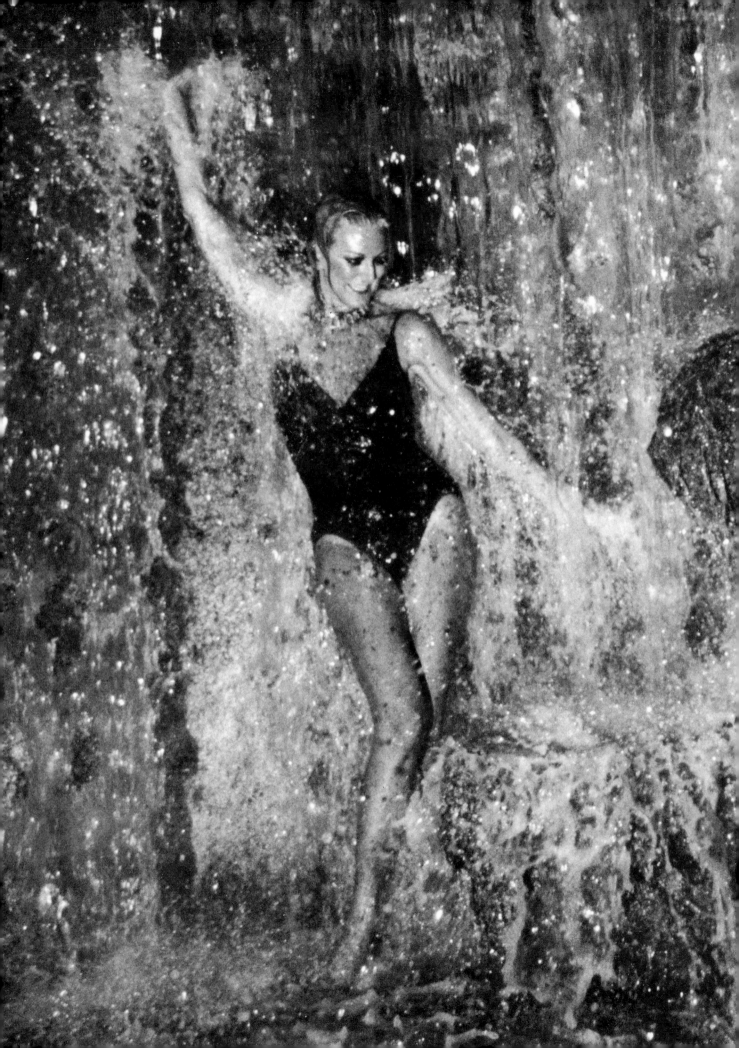

3

---※---

EXERCISE

XERCISE IS THE OPPOSITE of eating candy. One piece of candy every now and then won't do anybody any harm, and fifteen minutes of exercise every now and then won't do anybody any good. More than that, we seem to have been born with a taste for sweets, but exercise is usually an acquired taste. Unless we've been doing it all our lives, it is very difficult to work up real enthusiasm for it, but no inner or outer health and beauty are possible without developing that enthusiasm. I love it. In addition to all of the good it does for my body, it gives me a sense of inner well-being, of calm and satisfaction, that sets me up for the rest of the day.

Exercise will redistribute weight, but it will not take weight off; burning up enough calories

to lose just one pound takes more physical activity than any of us are capable of at any one time. What exercise will do is use the nutrients we consume to build muscle and connective tissue instead of fat. We diet to lose weight, but we exercise to apportion our weight in the healthiest and most aesthetically pleasing way.

If you have not been exercising regularly, it is essential that you see a doctor before you begin. Check out your blood, heart, and lungs. Take a stress test to find out what your endurance and capacities are, and never try to push your body to a point beyond what it is capable of doing with only a small amount of extra effort. Little by little, that capacity will expand, but pushing beyond the limit at the beginning is more dangerous than helpful. There is only one rule: Reach that limit and don't stop before you get there because of boredom, or laziness, or even an occasional aching muscle. That ache is usually the muscle complaining you've awak-

---

I was born an air sign but have a natural affinity with water. *(Norman Parkinson)*

83

ened it from a deep and long sleep.

Let's define a regular regimen of exercise in terms of what it is *not*. It is not a Saturday morning tennis game, a winter ski jaunt, a summer weekend swim, a walk around the block, a sporadic exercise or dance class, a weekly visit to the gym. A regimen is a set of specific physical exertions performed at least three times a week and preferably every single day.

The best regimen is one designed to build strength, agility, coordination, endurance, and balance.

Strength is the amount of exertion your muscles can make.

Agility is the ease with which they function.

Coordination is the speed with which they respond to the brain's command.

Endurance is the ability to withstand stress.

Balance in this case is the harmony between outer activity and a sense of inner well-being.

If a regimen increases all of these faculties, it will also redefine the body's silhouette.

The link between physical health and exercise is a well-established one. Exercise will not only help you to look better, it will probably help you to look better longer by lengthening your life. The heart is the most important muscular organ in the body, and a good regimen practiced diligently will strengthen it and reduce the risk of heart disease. It will improve respiration and circulation by increasing the lungs' ability to process air, which adds to the amount of oxygen in the blood. Oxygen-rich blood means a more alert and healthy brain.

A sounder heart and brain, self-esteem, stamina, physical attractiveness, and strength—all of these can be obtained simply by following an exercise regimen. One might almost think of it as the greatest wonder drug in the world. Perhaps it is. It certainly has improved the quality of my life. At fourteen, I was that proverbial eighty-pound weakling. At fifty-four, I'm one of the healthiest and strongest people I know.

Certainly, Dr. Ogden's vitamin and hormone shots helped me along the way, but all of that increased weight would have gone to fat were it not for exercise. My mainstay of swimming, along with the exercises to which I was first introduced by Nicholas Kounovsky, are responsible for the lean and robust woman I am today.

There is an exercise regimen to suit almost anyone's needs and personality—and pocketbook, too, for some of them can get expensive. The important thing is to find the one that works best for you, and that you will work best at.

Most of us will find at least one exercise odious. In my case, it's jogging. Jogging is a perfectly good form of working out. It has gotten more people off their fannies and into shaping up than almost anything else that has come along in the last few years. It is reputedly wonderful for the heart, circulation, and respiratory system. It just doesn't do anything for me on a personal level. Perhaps it is because I live in a city and cannot believe that running along the streets and inhaling all that automobile exhaust is good for me. I also find it boring, and boredom is one of the most frequent reasons for putting off exercising. However, while the loneliness of the long-distance runner may not be for me, some of my friends do five miles a day and look and feel better than they did ten years ago.

Personally, I prefer long, brisk walks. They are as healthy as running and much more interesting because they give me the opportunity to really notice the world around me. Curiosity may kill a cat, but it's always made me feel more alive.

Exercise should turn you on as well as tune you up. There are wonderful alternatives for those who know they will never get on with it if they have to do it alone. Gymnastics, yoga, calisthenics, dance classes, and Nautilus-machine training programs are all beneficial group endeavors that become absolutely top-drawer regimens when performed three times a week. Their drawbacks are cost and time. They can be expensive, and you do have to travel to the places where the classes are given.

Golf has become a negligible form of exercise since the cart replaced the feet as the mode of transportation, but there are many sporting activities that do everything the sportswoman exerciser may require. These include bicycling, skiing, tennis, paddle ball, and swimming, but only if they remain sporting and not social events. The occasional endeavor with friends will do no good. Three sessions a week is a minimum for the proper results.

My day begins with exercise. I start before I get out of bed with three minutes of simple stretch exercises that get the circulation moving and tone the muscles.

This is actually a gentle sit-up. You are awakening your body with a healthy stretch.

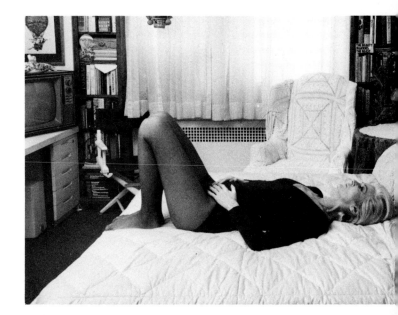

1. Start in a relaxed position with knees up and hands on your stomach. Breathe naturally a few times.

2. On an inhale, contract your stomach muscles, pulling the pelvis forward (this relieves undue pressure on the lower back). Rise slowly, pushing your hands out in front of you and lifting your feet off the bed. If necessary, pause to breathe on the rise, always moving on the exhale.

Inhale and return to the starting position. Repeat. Do this as often as you can, starting with two times and working up to ten.

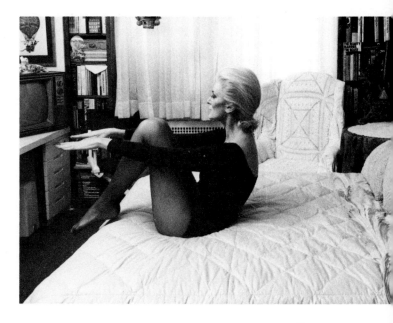

This one is slightly more strenuous.

1. Start in a sitting position with your hands under your thighs. On the exhale, slowly lift your legs with toes pointed out.

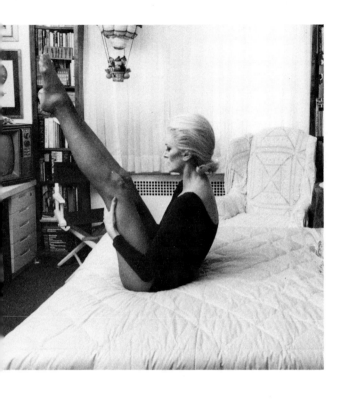

2. When legs are straight up, breathe a few times.

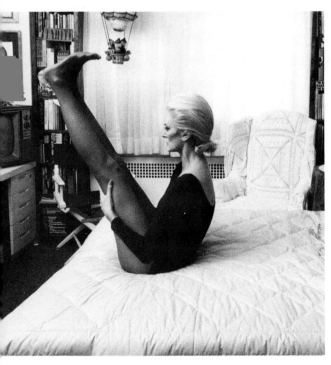

3. On the exhale, curl your toes toward your nose. Inhale and return to the starting position. Repeat.

This is one of the few exercises in which the exertion is on the inhale. You are filling your body with oxygen, which is so important for the system in the morning.

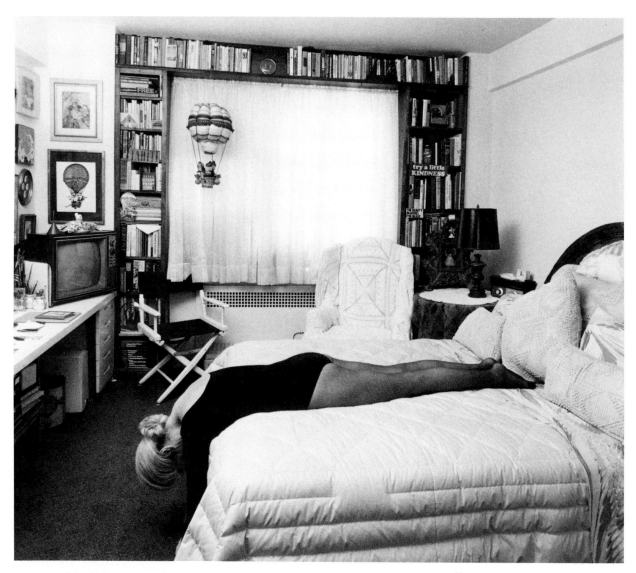

1. Lie on your stomach with arms extended over the edge of the bed and head down. The whole body should be relaxed with toes pointed out.

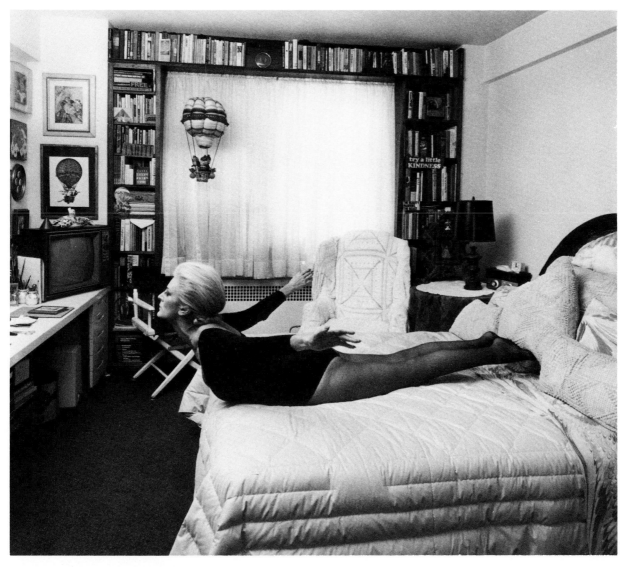

2. On the inhale, tighten your buttocks and stomach and arch your body as if doing a swan dive, lifting both head and toes.

Breathe, and on the exhale, return to starting position. Repeat.

Once I'm out of bed, the bedroom chair provides all of the equipment I need for my next wake-up exercises.

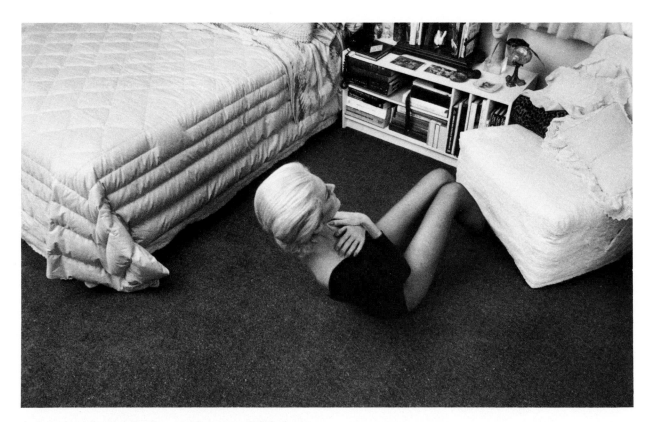

1. Start by lying on the floor with knees slightly bent, toes tucked under a chair, and arms crossed on your chest. Exhale, contracting your stomach muscles and pulling your pelvis forward. Rise slowly.

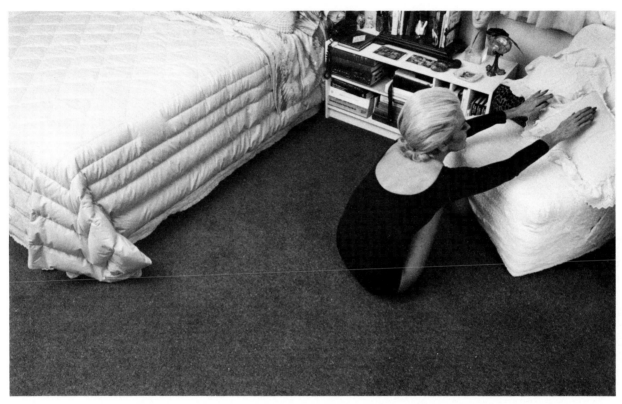

2. Extend your hands across the seat of the chair.
Inhale and on the exhale, return to the starting position.

This is the greatest stretch for the buttocks and wonderful for the neck and breasts as well.

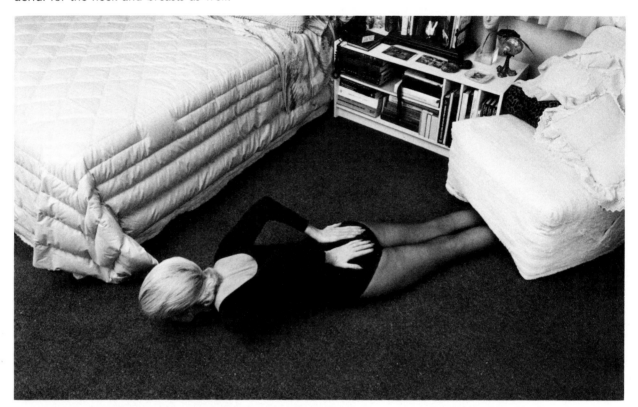

1. Lie on your stomach with feet under a chair, chin on the ground, hands on buttocks with elbows pointed up and close together. Inhale and lift chin up.

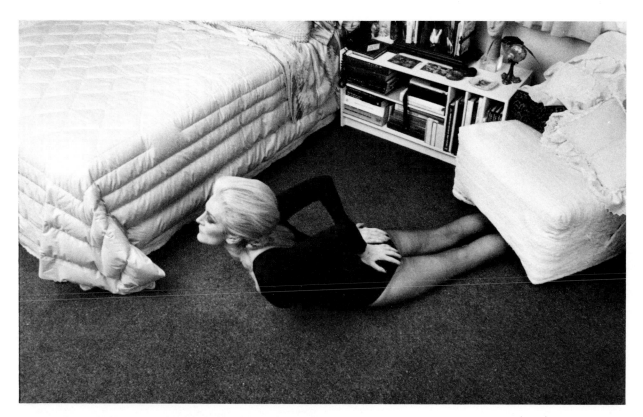

2. On the exhale, press down on the buttocks and
bring your head all the way up, lifting your chest off
the floor at the same time.

I have a bar in the frame of the bedroom door. Before I go to the kitchen to prepare breakfast, I swing from it. I do this several times during the day as I enter and leave the room. I can literally feel my body elongating and all of the kinks disappearing.

That bar in the bedroom doorframe is the world's greatest aid to stretching, whether swinging from side to side or right up off the ground.

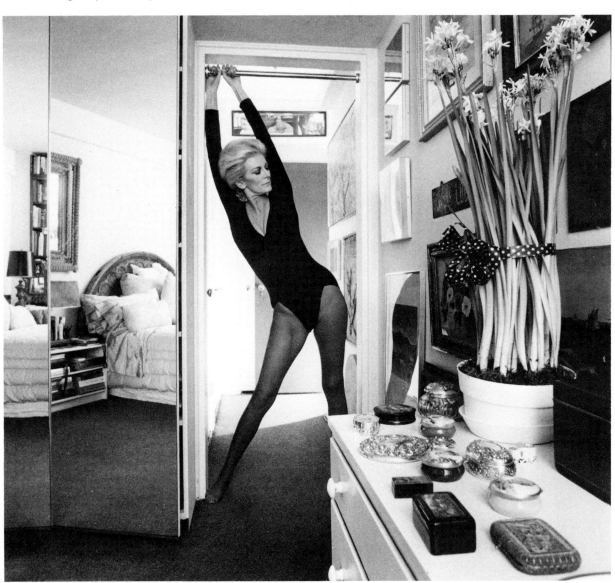

94

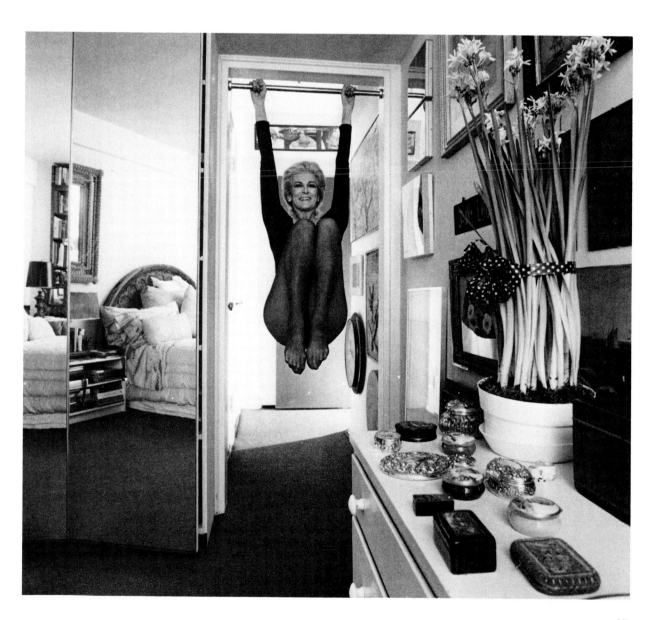

At my age, I find the most satisfying exercises are those based on the aerobic stretch. They are not too strenuous and they fit the schedule imposed by my career. I love to go to classes, but I don't have the time to do so often enough to get the full benefit out of them. My stretches can be done at home, in a hotel room on location, on a beach, or in a photographer's studio during the long waits that sometimes occur during a sitting.

My figure has the same trouble spots that beset any woman of my age: the waist, hips, backside, bust, thighs, and upper arms. When I don't exercise, they droop, sag, and get flabby. My stretches take care of all of those areas as well as stimulating the important organs inside my body.

I've already described how I rev up my body and circulation each day. Three times a week, I add fifteen minutes of other stretch exercises. I don't do the same ones for more than a month at a time. I rotate them because, to me, variety in exercise is as important as it is in any other part of my life. If there's anything that is self-defeating, it is that attitude of "Ho-hum, I've got to touch my toes ten times again. What a bore. I think I'll skip it today."

Aerobic literally means requiring the presence of air or oxygen for life. Proper breathing is as much a part of these exercises as are the stretches. It's very easy to master. With most exercises, the trick is to inhale before you start, exhale on the exertion, and inhale again on the release. For example, in touching your toes, you would take a deep breath, let it out as you lowered your arms, and breathe in again as you raised them.

Stretching is more strenuous than it looks. Start slowly, doing each exercise no more than two or three times and building slowly to ten. You will begin to get a feeling of physical well-being almost immediately. You will probably find you sleep more soundly and are able to accomplish more during the day without getting fatigued. But don't expect instantaneous visible change in the appearance of your body. It will happen, but, as in all exercise regimens, it will take time, patience, and faithful adherence to a schedule. The wonderful thing is that while you are waiting for the new outer look of you, you will be building inner stamina and health.

The human body is the greatest machine the world has ever known. Like most machines, however, it is constantly battling against the pull of gravity, and years of this struggle cause a problem with alignment: The body is no longer erect, it is not centered, and the balance is off. The wonderful added benefit of aerobic stretches is that they realign the body with the forces of gravity, recentering it and restoring the balance that enables us to walk erectly and with pride, or, as they used to say in westerns, "walk tall," no matter what our actual height may be.

Even if an aerobic stretch exercise is designed primarily to help one area of the body, it generally has auxiliary advantages for other areas. Each is as close to a total exercise as one can get. Stretching is reaching. What I love about these exercises is the feeling they give me of constantly reaching for the attainable goal of lasting fitness.

To get the most out of aerobic stretches, there are some general rules that have to be observed.

1. Always start from a position of total relaxation.
2. Take a few deep breaths and visualize exactly where you want your body to go. Always keep an image in your mind of the optimal position.
3. Start slowly and build. Never try to push your body beyond its capacities.
4. If you feel a cramp in any part of your body, do not fight it. Stop immediately. Get yourself into a comfortable position. Relax, and allow your body to seek its center of gravity. Start to breathe deeply and very slowly. In-

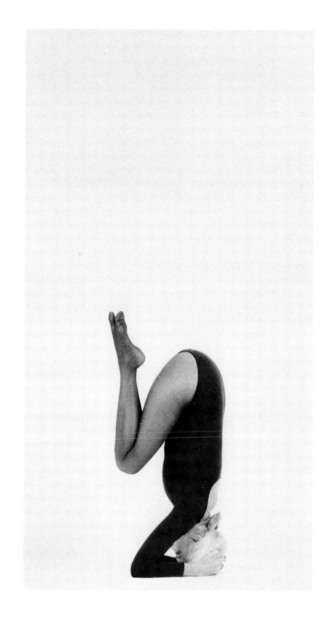

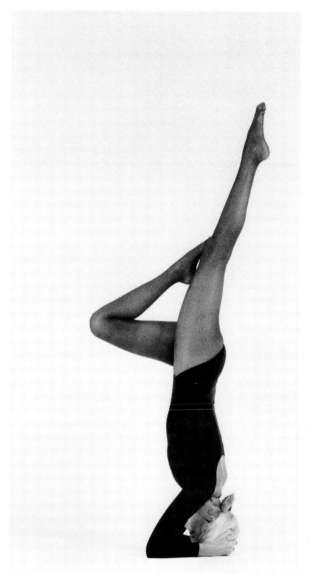

hale to the count of three and exhale to the count of three, and again visualize the optimal position. If the cramp persists, eliminate the exercise for the day.

Many of these exercises can be done with hand, wrist, or ankle weights. Use the weights only where you think you need extra help. If the problem is the upper arms or breasts, hand weights will help. If the problem is the legs, ankle weights can be added. But *never start your regimen with weights.* They should not be added until you have been doing the exercise for at least six months. Actually, if you do your exercises correctly and slowly, you usually do not need weights. You are not pumping iron; you are doing aerobic stretches.

There are three positions from which one starts to exercise: upright; prone; in a crouch. Because I find it logical to do them in sequence, I'm going to give all of the upright exercises first, followed by the reclining ones, and ending with the crouch.

UPRIGHT

EXERCISE 1

For the Waistline

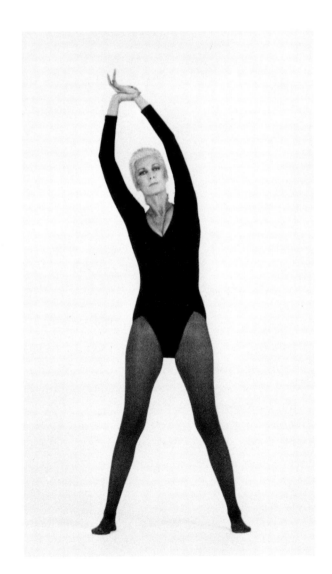

1. Stand with your legs apart. Your weight should be evenly distributed on the outer sides of your feet to give you better balance. Place your hands above your head with your right hand grasping your left wrist, again for balance. Take a few deep breaths.

98

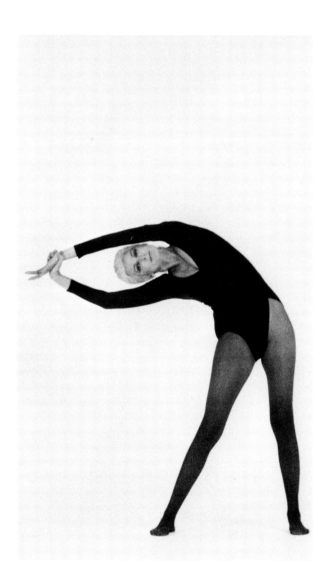

2. On an exhale, contract your buttock muscles and thrusting the pelvis forward, start to lower your body to the right. See how far down you can get. If necessary, stop to take a breath, moving again on the exhale. The breathing must be deep. If you feel light-headed, stop and start again. The light-headedness is only because you are not used to such deep breathing. Do not pull your body down by the hand grasping the wrist. The torso must do all the work.

When you are down as far as you can go, inhale and start up. You will almost seem to be floating up.

Grasp your right wrist with your left hand and repeat to the other side. Breathe deeply, relax into the stretch, always moving slowly, always keeping that pelvis slightly thrust forward and the buttocks contracted.

EXERCISE 2

For the Waistline

This is a more strenuous version of Exercise 1.

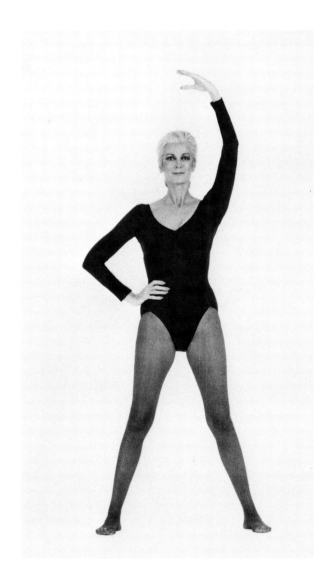

1. Again, the legs are apart with the weight on the outsides of the feet. The right hand is on the hip and the left above the head.

100

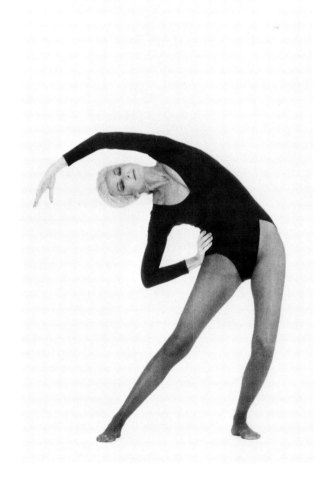

2. On the exhale, push your right hip sideways to the left with your hand, and as you start to lower the trunk to the right, bend your left knee and drop your head down to the right as if trying to touch your shoulder with your ear. Pause for as many breaths as you need, always moving on the exhale. Get down as far as you can. This has to be done very slowly.

Rise on the inhale and repeat with the left hand on the hip.

EXERCISE 3

For the Waistline and Lower Back Tension

Do not do this exercise if you have a back problem.
This is a good one to do with weights when and if you are ready to use them. Weights should weigh no more than 2 to 5 pounds. They bring added benefits to the upper arms and bust.

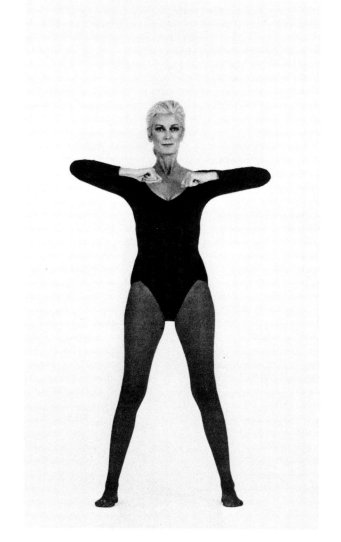

1. The legs are apart with the weight on the outer sides of the feet. With your fists clenched and pointing toward your chest and your elbows raised to shoulder-level, contract your stomach and buttock muscles. The pelvis is pushed forward and acts as the pivot on which the torso turns, first to the right and then to the left.

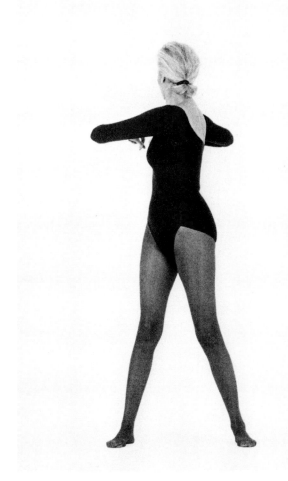

2. The object is to try to look at the wall behind you without moving either feet or head. Exhale on the turn to the back and inhale on the return to the front.

For Legs from Toes to Buttocks

This exercise helps prevent stiffening and arthritic problems in the toes, feet, and ankles. You may have some trouble with balance when you first start to do this exercise. If you do, it will help if you focus on a point in front of you.

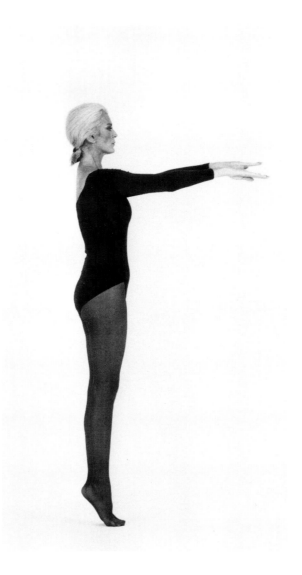

1. Start from a completely relaxed stance, feet flat on the ground, arms stretched out in front of you. Take a few deep breaths. On the exhale, squeeze your buttocks together, pull the pelvis forward, and rise on the balls of your feet. Hold the position for a count of three, then lower the heels on the inhale.

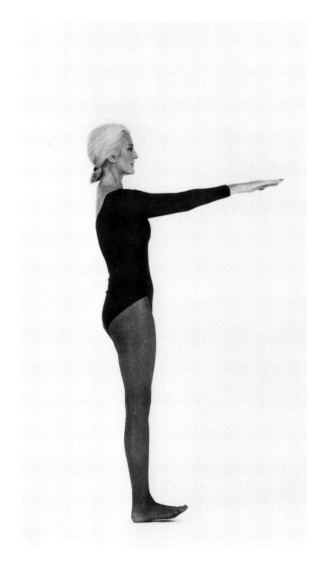

2. Breathe a few times and, on the exhale, raise your toes up off the floor, balancing on your heels. Hold for a count of three, and lower your toes on the inhale.

105

For Thighs, Calves, and Breasts

Another good exercise with weights.

1. With legs apart, bend forward at the waist thrusting buttocks back. Keep your chin high. Raise your elbows, keeping them close to the body, and bring your fists close to the shoulders.

2. Exhale and slowly bring your arms straight out behind you feeling the stretch in your upper arms. Take a few breaths. Keep chin raised high.

Inhale, and slowly return to Position 1.

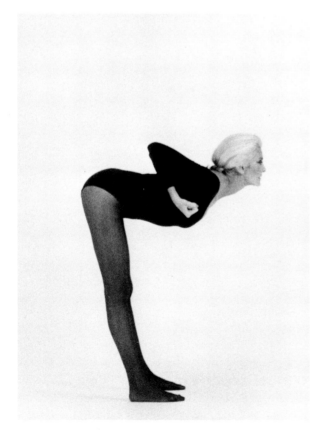

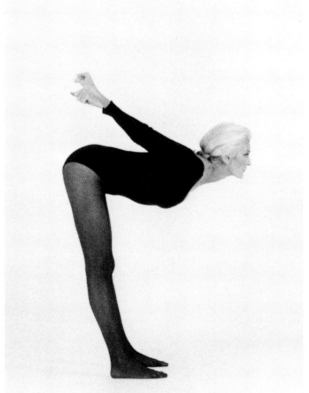

For Upper Arms

A very good exercise with weights. In the photographs, I am using a roll of paper towels in place of a 2-pound weight.

1. Stand with your feet together. Raise hands above the head with elbows close to the head.

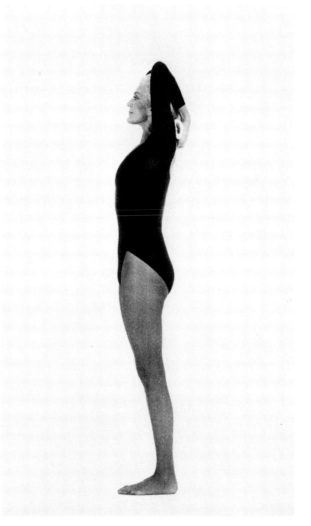

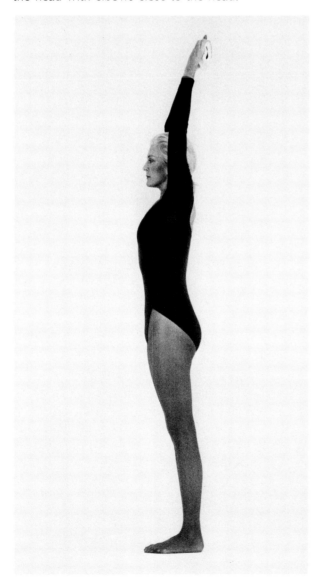

2. On the exhale, pull the pelvis forward and lower the hands behind your head, focusing on pulling your elbows back behind your ears while keeping them close to the head as your hands reach the back of your neck. Take a few breaths and relax your body.

On the inhale, relax the pelvis and raise your arms above your head again. Repeat.

107

For Upper Arms, Breasts

In this exercise, there must be isometric tension. If you are doing it correctly, you feel tension in the upper arm. Your breasts are also getting the benefit of the stretch. While raising your arms, you are pushing against gravity and oxygenating the entire body by taking in all the air you can as you stretch.

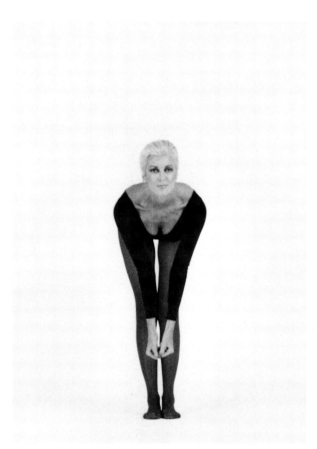

1. With legs close together and straight, bend forward at the waist, thrusting your buttocks back. Focus on a point in front of you, keeping your chin high, and arms hanging down in front of you with fists clenched. (If you use a weight, so much the better).

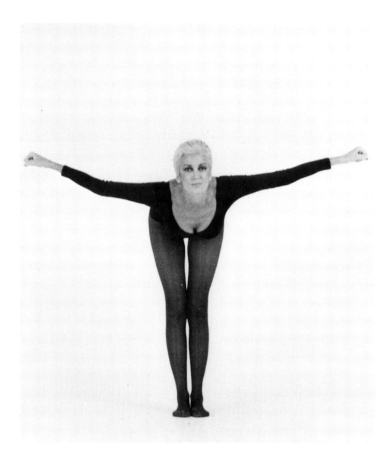

2. The breathing is reversed in this exercise. You inhale
and stretch the arms up to the side—*stretch,* not raise
or lift.

Exhale and lower your arms.

Repeat.

For Thighs and Buttocks

This exercise is a good test of balance and harder to do than it may look. It will take time to get it right, but it is worth it.

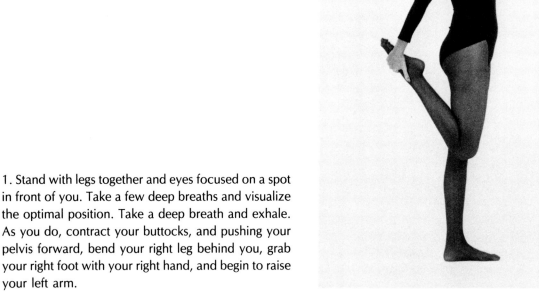

1. Stand with legs together and eyes focused on a spot in front of you. Take a few deep breaths and visualize the optimal position. Take a deep breath and exhale. As you do, contract your buttocks, and pushing your pelvis forward, bend your right leg behind you, grab your right foot with your right hand, and begin to raise your left arm.

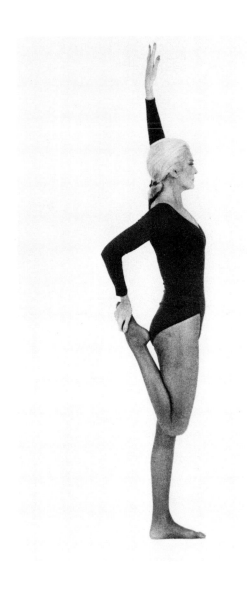

2. As you raise your left arm, bring the foot up as far as you can. Keep the elbow straight back; do not let it slip sideways. Perfection is when you can touch your buttock with your heel, with the left arm extended straight up. This may take some pauses for breath along the way.

Inhale, lower the foot, release it, and let it descend to the ground.

Take a few more deep breaths and repeat with the left foot.

EXERCISE 9

For Neck, Hips, Thighs, Abdomen

This is an easy exercise but it must be done slowly so that you feel the stretch.

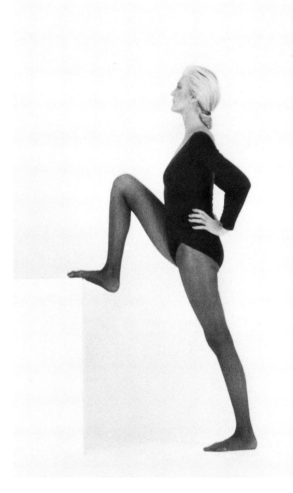

1. Place the ball of your right foot on the edge of a table. With your body as erect as possible and your hands on your hips, exhale and push the pelvis forward toward your raised heel.

112

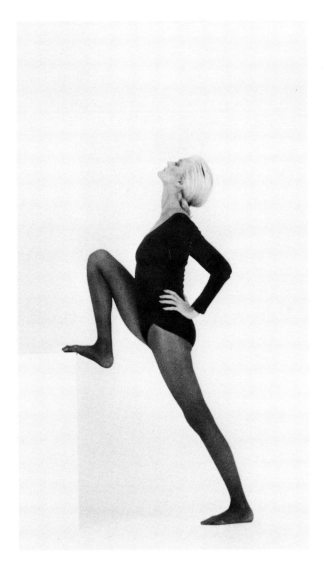

2. At the same time, push your head all the way back. Thrust forward with the pelvis but do not bend your knee. The head action is stimulating the thyroid and working on the neck muscles.

Inhale as you lower your head and relax the pelvis. Repeat with the left foot on the table.

For Legs, Abdomen, Balance

Balance is the tricky part of this exercise. If you have problems with it, you can rest your hands on the edge of a table instead of extending them in front of you. But do try to do it from a free-standing position.

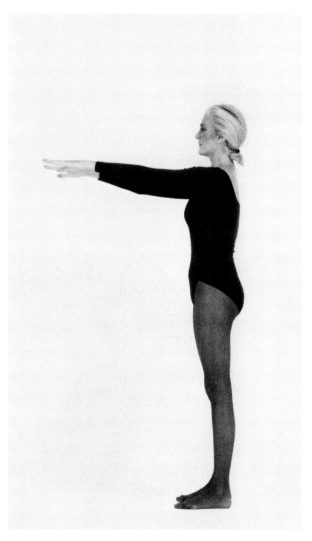

1. Start in a standing position, arms extended in front of you, pelvis thrust forward.

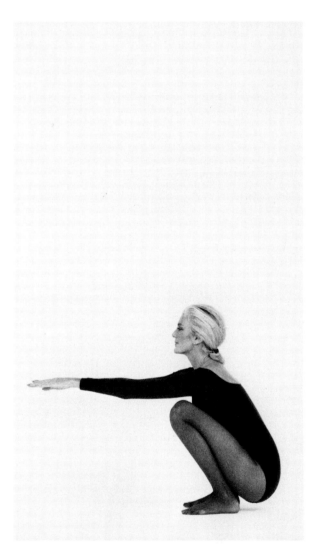

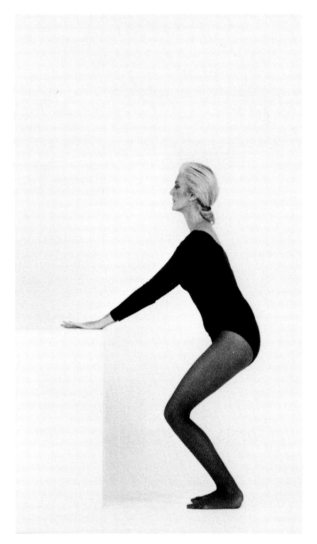

2. Exhale and lower your trunk to a full squat, keeping your heels flat on the ground at all times.

3. Inhale and rise. If you have to, take a few breaths on the way down. Pause and continue moving on the exhale.

For the Torso from Hips to Breasts to Arms

In exercises that entail touching your toes or the floor in front of you, the object is to think of lowering your head rather than stretching your arms. Let your body do the work, and the arms will lower by themselves. It is gravity again. You are going with it. The weight of your head going down will release the tension in the lower back muscles. The first few times you do it, you may not get all the way down. Don't worry about it —you will in time. If you get only as far your knees, do the pivot grasping your calves instead of your feet. If you do it correctly, this exercise can be a great relaxer. It stretches all the tensions out of the torso.

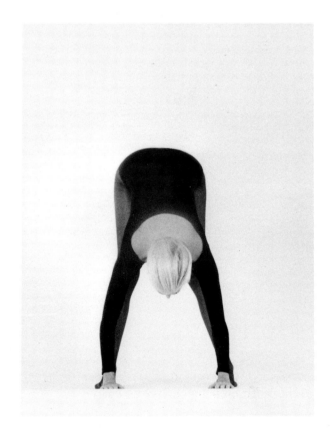

1. Start in a relaxed upright position, arms hanging loosely at sides, legs apart, weight on the outer sides of the feet. Breathe deeply and visualize the optimal position. Exhale with your chin tucked in toward the chest, letting the weight of the head pull the torso toward the floor as far down as you can go. Keep your shoulders relaxed and take several breaths. If you can touch the floor, take several breaths in this position.

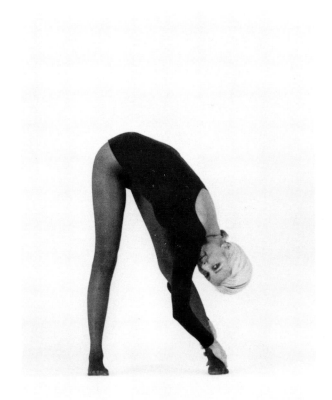

2. The whole body pivots on the hip as you reach first for the right foot and then the left, or that part of the opposite leg that is at hand level. You will feel the stretch from the heel, up the leg, through the hips, through the breasts, and to the upper arms.

Inhale and rise to a standing position.

EXERCISE 12

Total from Legs through Torso to Arms

This is a difficult exercise but a very rewarding one. Before you can do it, you must master touching the floor in front of your feet (see Exercise 11).

1. With your legs together, lower your arms until your hands are flat on the ground about 30 inches in front of you. Your body is forming a triangle with the ground, and your weight is evenly distributed between hands and feet. Keep your heels flat on the ground throughout.

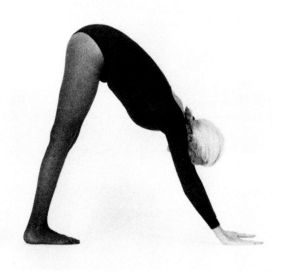

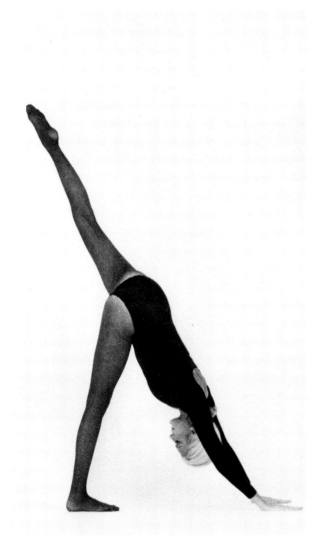

2. Exhale, press down on your hands and drop your head between your shoulders raising a leg out behind you. Breathe deeply and exhale as you extend the leg all the way up in the air. Your body should be a straight diagonal line from foot to hands. Take a few deep breaths, inhale, and lower your foot to the ground. Repeat with the other leg.

EXERCISE 13

For Thighs and Lower Back Tension

This is a great relaxer. Review Exercise 11 before start-ing. The starting position in this one is with the legs slightly apart with the knees relaxed. They must not be locked or rigid.

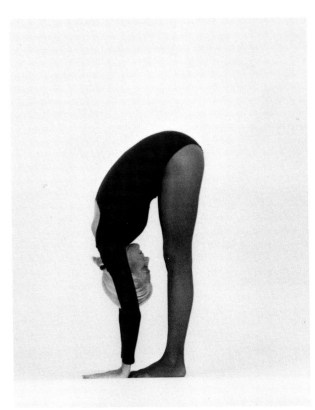

1. As your hands touch the floor, your head is between your arms and looking at your knees, which are relaxed and slightly bent. Breathe a few times. You will feel a release of the tension in the lower back.

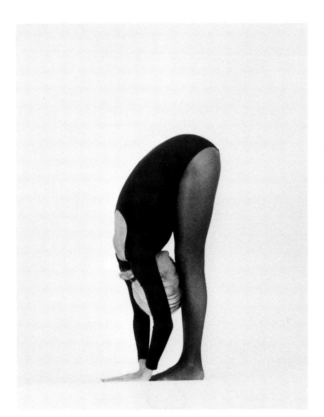

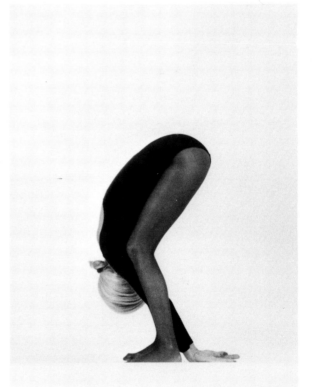

2. Tuck your chin in so that you are looking at your navel.

3. Breathe; bend your knees; and on the exhale, reach between your legs to touch the floor behind your feet with your palms up. Inhale and rise to the upright position. Repeat.

EXERCISE 14

For Calves and Inner Thighs

In this exercise, it is important to do your deep breathing before starting.

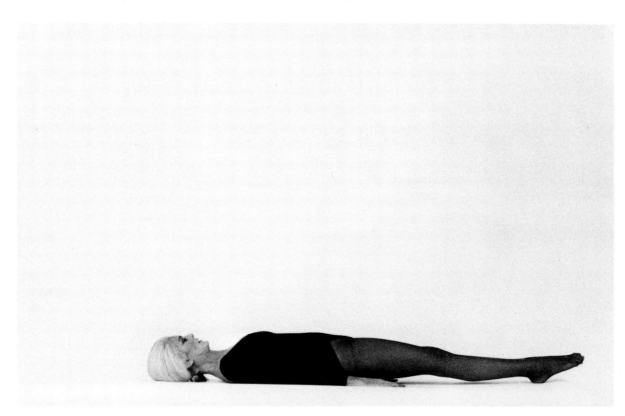

1. Recline on your back with your palms flat on the ground. Pull in your stomach so that all of the vertebrae are touching the ground.

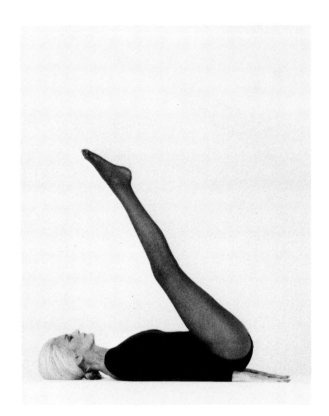

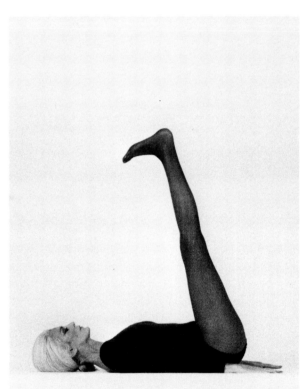

2. Exhale and, with toes pointed, raise your legs straight up. Your buttocks should be off the ground but your vertebrae still in contact with it.

3. Breathe and, on the exhale, turn your toes toward your head so that your feet are parallel to your body. Breathe. Inhale as you slowly lower your legs with toes pointed out. Relax and repeat.

For Thighs, Buttocks, Abdomen

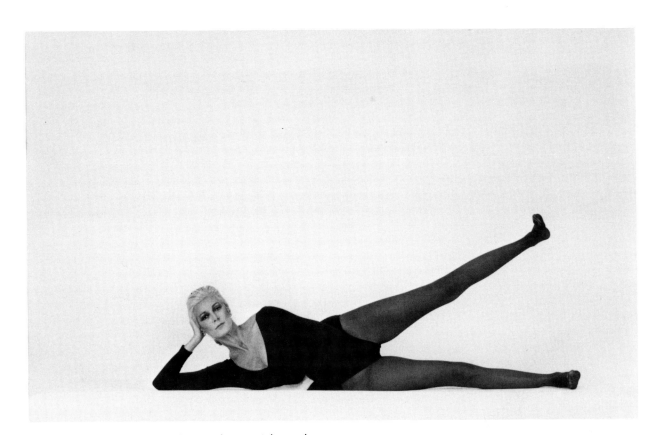

1. Recline on your side with your feet at right angles to your ankles. Support your head with your hand. The other hand is placed palm flat on the floor in front of you. Roll forward slightly, balancing your weight on the front hand. Breathe naturally during this exercise. Contract your stomach muscles and, with slightly squeezed buttocks, raise your leg about halfway up. Do not relax as you lower your leg. This must be done very slowly, going down until your foot almost but not quite touches your other foot. Repeat as often as you can and then switch sides to do the exercise with the other leg.

For Torso from Hips to Breasts and Upper Arms

In this exercise, if you change your foot position so that you do the exercise with toes pointed one time and pulled up the next, you will have a complete isometric stretch from toes to neck. It is a total exercise and very important. It is also very simple once you've mastered it.

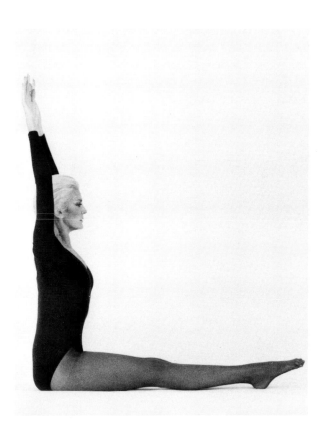

1. Sit up as erectly as you can, toes pointed out (as shown) or up. Raise your hands straight up with elbows pulled as far behind the ears as possible. Your body should form a perfect right angle.

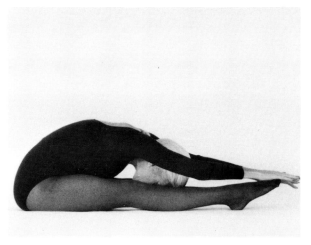

2. Exhale and lower your hands toward your toes. Think of yourself as lowering your chin to your knees rather than using your fingers to pull your body toward your toes. Try to get your fingers past your toes. You may not be able to do it at first, but keep trying. When you are down as far as you can go, take a deep breath and on the inhale, rise to the original position with your hands really stretching for the sky.

For Thighs and Abdomen

This is a very challenging exercise. It is not for beginners, but if you work up to it, it is very rewarding. It tones the muscles close to the bone on the outer side of the thigh, which is where fat gathers and sags when the muscles are lax.

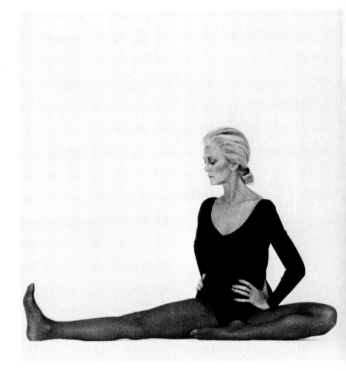

1. Stretch a leg out to one side with toes pointed up. Tuck the other leg up as close as possible to the torso. The thigh of this leg must at all times touch the ground. Place your hands on your hips and breathe, using the breathing time to focus on where you want your body to go.

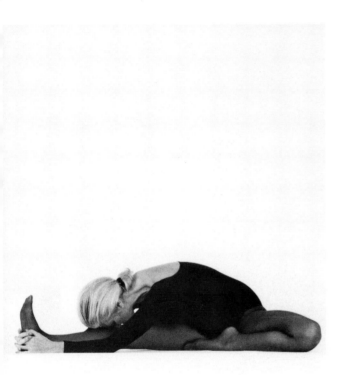

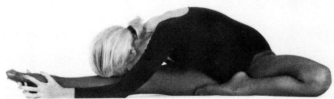

2. Using your hips as a pivot, turn the entire body toward the extended leg while keeping the other thigh in contact with the floor. Gently, slowly, pausing to breathe when necessary, moving on the exhale, lower your head toward your knee, extending your arms to try to loosely fold your hands around your heel.

3. Your knee is straight. Breathe; and on the exhale, with hands folded around the foot, point your toes out. Inhale and bring your toes back up, releasing the foot as you rise to a sitting position with your hands once more on your hips. Relax and repeat with the other foot.

For the Pelvic Area and Thighs

For this exercise, it is best to keep your legs together, but beginners will find it easier and still derive a good deal of the benefit if they keep their legs apart.

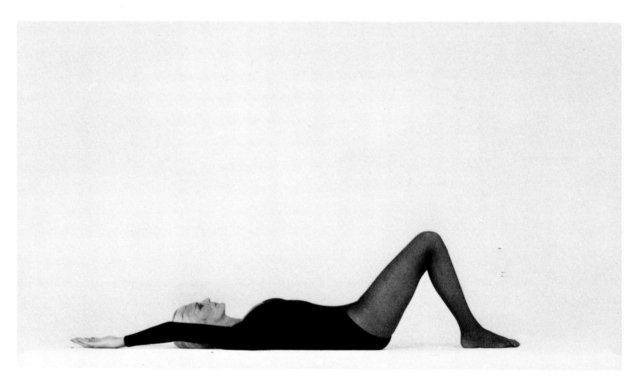

1. Reclining with your arms stretched over your head, palms up, and your knees bent, do your heavy breathing and visualizing.

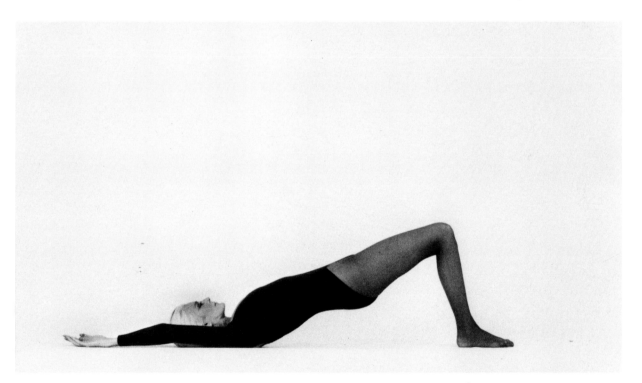

2. Keep your buttocks tight, exhale, press down on your feet, and contracting your stomach muscles, thrust up as far as you can. You may have to pause to breathe on the way up, but, as usual, move on the exhale.

Take a few breaths, inhale, and lower your body. Relax and repeat.

For Abdomen, Backs of Thighs, Balance

This is a good exercise for ankle or wrist weights, or both. They extend the benefits respectively to the calves and bust.

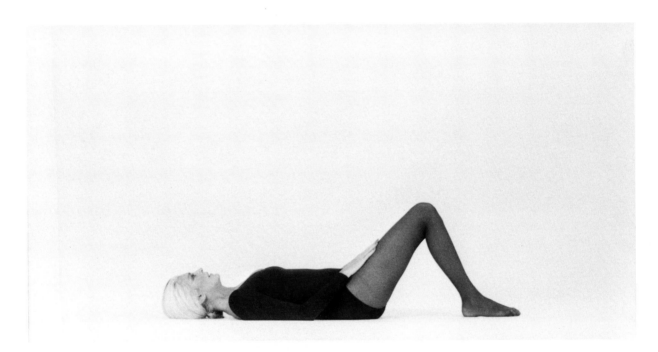

1. Lie on your back with knees bent and hands resting on thighs.

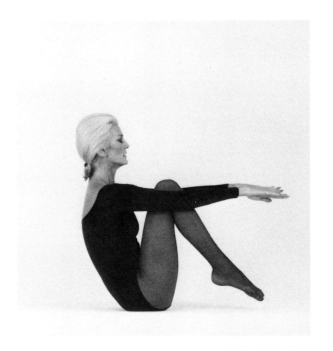

2. Exhale and raise your torso, balancing on your buttocks, and simultaneously extend your arms forward. Keep your chin raised at all times. Lift your feet off the ground. By this time, you should need to inhale again.

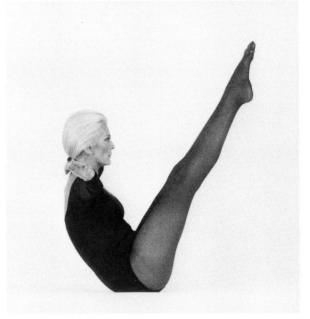

3. On the exhale, spread your arms out to your sides and, contracting your stomach muscles, lift your feet straight up in front of you. A few more breaths and, on the exhale, return to Position 2 with arms extended in front of you and feet off the ground.

A few more breaths and, on the inhale, return to the starting position.

Relax and repeat.

131

For Abdomen, Thighs, and Hips

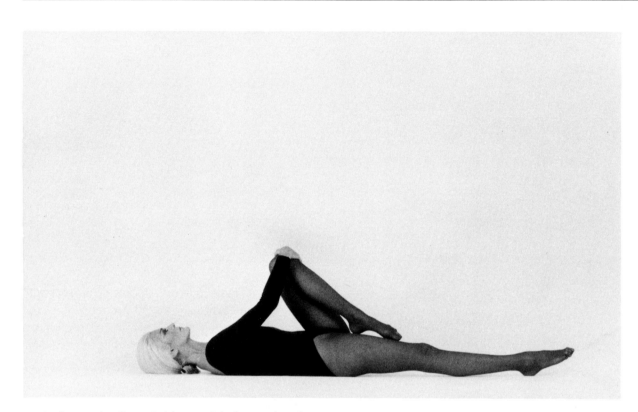

1. Lie flat on the floor. Fold your right leg so that the calf is as close as possible to the back of the thigh with the foot resting lightly on the other thigh. Take hold of the knee with your hands.

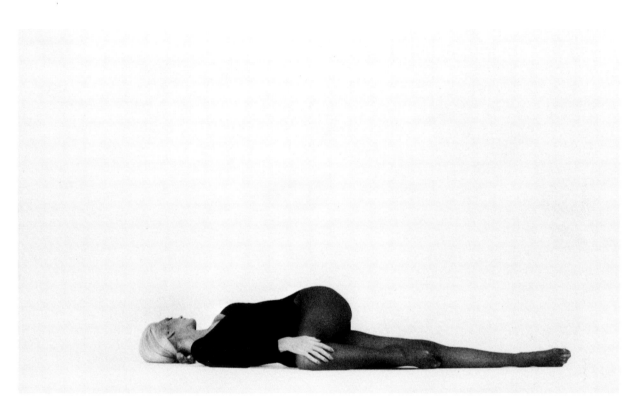

2. Exhale and lower the knee to the left till it touches the floor. Turning your head in the opposite direction at the same time gives added benefits to the chin, jawline, and neck.

Inhale and bring your leg back up.

Slowly return to a completely supine position and repeat with the other leg.

CROUCH

The Two-in-One

This simple and extremely effective exercise is called the "two-in-one" because the first part is excellent for the neck, chin, and jawline, and the second part is wonderful for the abdomen, shoulders, breasts, and upper arms.

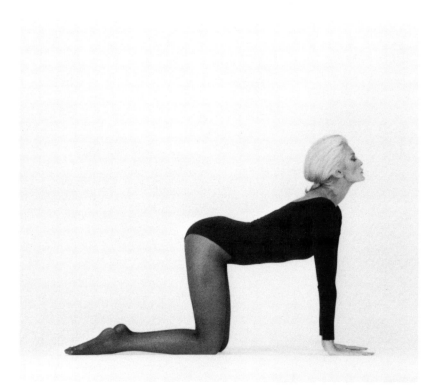

1. Start on your hands and knees. Your trunk, thighs, and arms should form a square with the floor. Breathe a few times. On the inhale, raise your head as high as you can. Do some really heavy breathing, inhaling with your mouth wide open and closing it as you exhale. Do this at least three times.

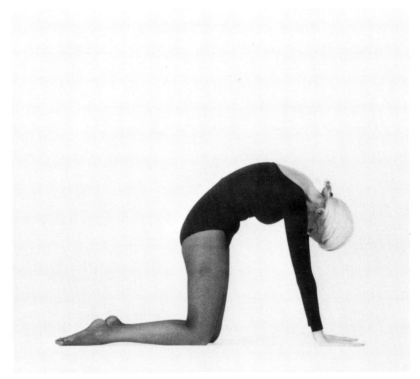

2. On the inhale again, lower your head until it is almost between your shoulders. Breathe a few times and, on the exhale, contract your stomach muscles and pull up, rolling your back into an arch from the bottom vertebrae to the neck. Breathe and, on the inhale, relax. Repeat as often as you need to achieve a state of relaxation along the vertebrae from the shoulders to the lower back.

EXERCISE 22

For Tension in the Neck and Shoulders

I think of this as the stretch that saves my life. I have
a little arthritis in my neck, and when I'm tense I get
terrible knots in my shoulders. One of the loving
chores of my husbands was to massage that part of my
body. Now that I'm alone, this exercise takes their
place.

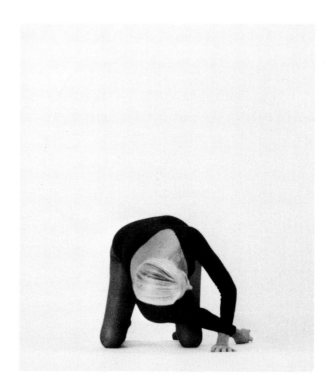

1. Start with the body in the square of Exercise 21.
Breathe a few times and thread your right arm through
the space between the left arm and your thigh.

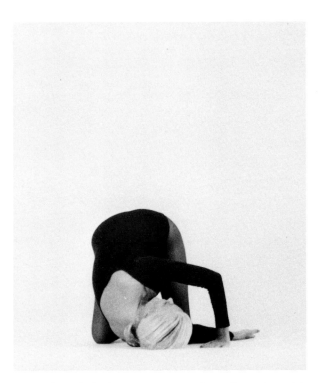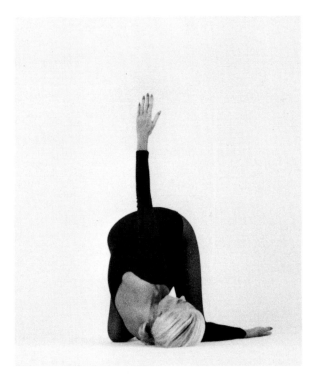

2. On the exhale, lower your torso from the waist, with hips raised. Slowly lower your head until the right shoulder and the right side of your head are firmly resting on the floor.

3. Take deep breaths and turn your chin as far toward the ceiling as possible, pressing down on the floor with the left palm. With all your weight supported by the right shoulder and head, lift your left arm. It should feel almost weightless in space. If your ears pop, don't worry about it.

Breathe a few times. On the exhale, bring your left arm back down. Shift your weight to it. On the inhale, push down, and you should really float up.

Repeat with the other arm.

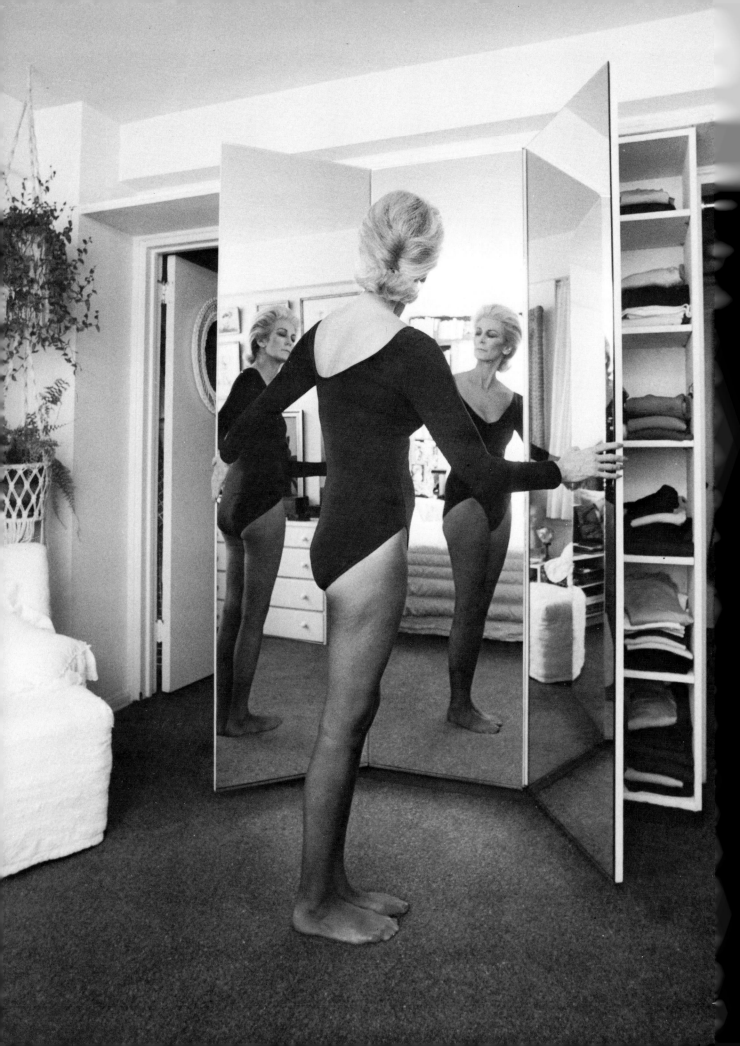

4

DIET

DIET HAS BECOME ONE OF the nastiest words in the English language because of connotations that have nothing to do with its definition. It is not a painful ordeal designed to put on or take off weight except in the narrowest sense. A diet is everything we eat and drink considered in terms of its quality and effect on our health. It is the fuel that keeps our bodies, brains, and, yes, our emotions running. The better the quality of that fuel, the more likely we are to become the healthy, vital, alert, alluring, sexual creatures of our aspirations. Let us consider *diet* in the largest rather than the most constricting sense of the word.

Achieving our ideal selves must start with a recognition of where we are in our lives. Food extremism is bad at any age, but at ours it is completely self-defeating and will never win our objectives of harmony, balance, and glowing good health. Food fetishes and fad or crash diets will often leave us in worse shape than they found us. Calories do count, so do carbohydrates, fats, and proteins. There is no such thing as a "quickie" seven-day or twenty-one-day diet that will help anybody except the author/expert, who will probably earn a lot of money on it. Those fellows (and most of them *are* fellows) are more concerned with their fat bankrolls than our fat middles. To put it simply, the only diet that works for the rest of your life is a balanced diet. It is also the only painless diet, and the only one that is as good for the spirit as it is for the flesh. In our culture and at our age, it is impossible not to overindulge at one moment or another, and we're much better off enjoying the pleasurable experience rather than doing penance for it. If our diet is balanced, we can make up for the splurge by only

It's harder to deceive yourself in a three-way mirror.

the slightest amount of abstinence spread over the following few days.

It's been said often enough that inside every fat woman, there's a thin woman longing to get out. I don't think that's necessarily true. I know a lot of very happy large women who think of thin as some kind of nervous disease. Let's take a closer look at that ultraslim, very "in" lady. We've all seen her. She watches every morsel she eats and exercises to a fare-thee-well, and yet she often projects a restless unhappiness. Despite her wonderful figure, carefully made-up face, and trendy clothes, her compulsive talking, moodiness, lack of repose, and egocentricity combine to make her a quite unattractive companion. What she seems unaware of is that the central nervous system also requires a carefully balanced diet, that flexibility and harmony are the cornerstones of beauty and not a lithe body or perfect coiffure. She makes me wonder if it might not be true that inside many thin women, there are fat ones longing to get out.

The latest studies indicate that people tend to be healthier and live longer if they weigh slightly more than the "ideal" weights given in the charts that appear in diet and exercise books. If a woman "should" weigh 125 pounds and tips the scale at about 130, she may actually be in better shape, so long as those extra five pounds are not pure fat. She must have the proper diet, and she must exercise.

The woman with a tendency to overweight must beware of obesity, which is defined as 20 percent above the norm. Our 125-pound example becomes obese at 145 or over. At that point, she is endangering her health, and slimming down is absolutely necessary.

There are equal dangers at the other end of the scale. If she gets down closer to 100 pounds, she is in danger of developing pernicious anemia as well as becoming prey to the entire range of contagious diseases. Being too thin can also be very bad for the skin of a woman in the balanced years. The layer of subcutaneous fat beneath the dermis provides elasticity and youthfulness. If a woman gets too thin at exactly the age when the skin is beginning to lose its vitality, she is doubling the problem by diminishing the subcutaneous fat. The result often is early wrinkles, crepiness, and sags.

The decision to lose or gain weight should depend on only two factors: health and self-image. In any instance in which ten or more pounds is involved, a physician should be consulted before changing one's diet. When losing weight is the objective, all fad and crash diets must be avoided. I have a general rule: Easy-go weight loss is easy-return weight gain. In fact, crash diets make us lose muscle first and fat later—exactly the opposite of the gains we want to be making. And when we're crash dieting, the body burns the calories more slowly than usual, with all that effort not really counting for much in the way of results.

All diets must be accompanied by exercise. Only exercising will indicate to the body where we want the change in dimension. If we're gaining, we want to gain muscle rather than excess fatty tissue. If we're losing, we want to lose in the right place and to strengthen the muscles that will prevent any fleshy sag.

Your silhouette should not be subject to the whim of fashion or the opinions of friends. If you are in good health, only your eye and the mirror should dictate your shape. Once the decision to change is made, there are a few general rules I recommend you follow:

- Gain or lose as gradually as possible.
- Weigh yourself only once a week. If you do it more often on a gradual regime, the slowness of results will be discouraging.
- Try not to tell friends or family that you are dieting. When we are on a diet, some psychological quirk makes even those who love us most try to force the wrong foods on us.
- Make a fixed number of calories your goal for the week instead of the day, so that if

you fall off your diet on one day, you can compensate over the next few days.

- Never allow yourself to feel hunger pangs. Drink a lot of water or munch on raw vegetables (always keeping track of the number of calories in them).
- Eat small portions of many foods rather than large portions of any single food.
- No alcoholic beverage (and that includes white wine, which is bad for the digestion and liver). Never think you can make up for the 150 calories in a drink by skipping 150 calories of something else. Alcohol contains no essential nutrients, so by skipping the calories in another item in order to drink, you are also eliminating necessary vitamins and minerals.
- Eat as much fiber and bran as possible. Diets tend to constipate, and fibers are nature's own laxative.
- If your body sends out a message that it needs energy in the form of something sweet, listen to it. Have a piece of fruit, a glass of orange juice, even a small dish of plain ice cream. If the message is sent too often, don't listen. It is probably not coming from your body but from some self-destructive part of your psyche.
- Keep careful track of any changes in your skin, hair, and nails. These are symptomatic of an unbalanced diet in which they are not being fed those things necessary for their health.
- Consume only one-fourth the amount of salt you normally consume. Salt causes liquid retention, and most of our excess weight is liquid. It is also linked to hypertension and stroke. We all need some salt or our bodies will dehydrate, but less than one-twentieth of an ounce per day will suffice.
- Try to keep to three balanced meals a day with no snacking in between. A large breakfast is better for you than a large dinner, because you need all the energy you can get when starting the day and do not digest your food as well in slumber at the end of it.

If you want to take off or put on only a few pounds, you can devise your own diet, which will be far healthier for you than any "quick" diet. By the time you're finished, you will probably find you have also begun to form new eating habits, and that is the only way to make certain you never have to gain or lose again. This diet will also serve as a standard for the way you eat for the rest of your life. It is based on a very simple mathematical formula.

From grade school on, we've learned about the three essential nutrients: proteins, fats, and carbohydrates. Not all of these nutrients are equal. There are good and bad examples of each. Any good book on nutrition will tell you all you have to know on the subject. It will also tell you about the vitamins and minerals you need and which foods contain them. The ideal food contains good doses of vitamins and minerals as well as the necessary nutrients. Vitamin and mineral pills will never substitute for the natural nutritional elements in what we eat when we eat properly.

When preparing our diets, it must be remembered that as we get older, what we eat should be divided into about 60 percent carbohydrates, 30 percent fats, and only 10 percent proteins. This statistic should be enough to keep you off low-carbohydrate/high protein diets, especially the ones that are also high in fat.

Once you know the proportion of nutrients, vitamins, and minerals and which foods give you the best value for the calories, we are ready to discuss quantities. All foods have calories, and the amount you eat should be measured in them. As I've said, calories do count, and unless you count them, you will never become the woman you want to be for the rest of your life. In these days of cockamamie diets, this may sound so reactionary that it's almost come round the full circle to being revolutionary, but it's the only foolproof way.

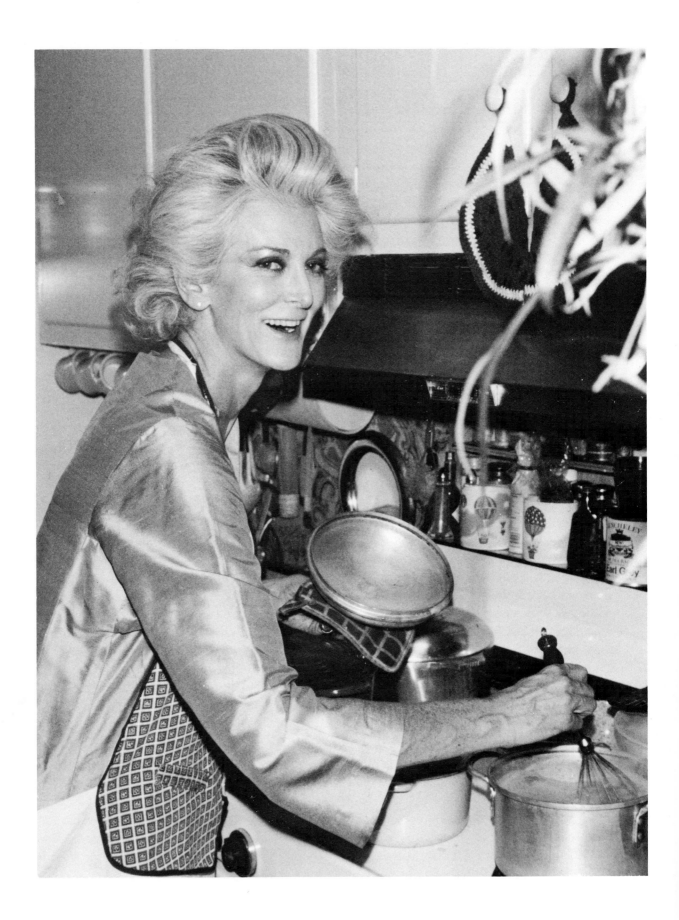

To maintain your weight, you should consume approximately fifteen calories per pound. Our 125-pound woman should restrict herself to 1,875 calories a day. If she overindulges one day, she should hold back over the next few days to regain her balance of 13,125 calories a week. Taking off those few calories a day should never be postponed to the point where it becomes a weight problem that is measured in pounds.

One pound of body fat adds up to 3,500 calories. It doesn't matter if the calories are taken in the form of scotch or celery, 3,500 extra calories a week will still put on one pound. Let's say our 125-pound friend has let herself go and gained five pounds. To lose them, she is going to have to cut back 17,500 calories. If she fasts for a week, she'll probably be almost back down to her normal weight. She'll also probably be hallucinating.

The very sensible and patient woman will restrict herself to her 1,875 calories a day, and in time she will return to 125 pounds. But it will take a long time, and most of us want quicker results. A cutback to 1,200 calories a day, 8,400 a week, will produce the desired weight loss in something less than three weeks. If those daily 1,200 calories are in the form of a balanced diet, it can also be the start of a balanced life with no more fears of what that weekly weigh-in will reveal. All she need do is retain the balance after she returns to her normal 1,875.

FOOD FOR BEAUTY. Our metabolisms change as we grow older. We also produce less estrogen. These two biological facts of older life combine to age our skin, hair, and nails—but there are foods that will help to strengthen and revitalize these areas.

Hair and nails are made of protein, hence an adequate supply will certainly help to enhance their quality. Most high-protein foods, however, also contain fat, and fat produces fat. Therefore, if you are increasing your fat intake for any reason, increase your level of activity and exercise.

In addition to protein, healthy nails need vitamins A and C, and iodine (from fish rather than salt).

Zinc and copper are two minerals extremely important to the hair. Inadequate zinc leads to hair loss, and a deficiency in copper causes accelerated depigmentation or graying.

Good skin requires that slight fatty subcutaneous layer. Green, leafy vegetables are a plus, and an adequate supply of water is a must. Actually, seven glasses of water a day will help keep the entire system in balance, because we eliminate so much liquid through the day and it must be replaced.

You should eat a sufficient amount of what are called "androgenic" foods. These include shellfish, wheat germ, gluten, liver, and kidneys. They contain high levels of androgen, a male sex hormone, or nutrients that have the same effect on the body's chemistry. Androgen stimulates the production of the oils that counteract skin dryness. These oils are secreted by the sebaceous glands, which begin to slow down as we get older.

If your complexion is important to you, there are certain things that are absolute "no-nos." Nicotine will cause dark circles under the eyes at just that time of life when nature is eroding that sensitive skin area. Alcohol, caffeine, and hot spices cause expansion of the blood vessels and eruption of the tiny capillaries on the cheeks and nose. The damage can become permanent with habitual imbibing of these nutritionally valueless substances. (For additional diet information, see chapter 6.)

I enjoy cooking for friends. This photograph was taken in the kitchen of my New York apartment. *(Sy Reisin)*

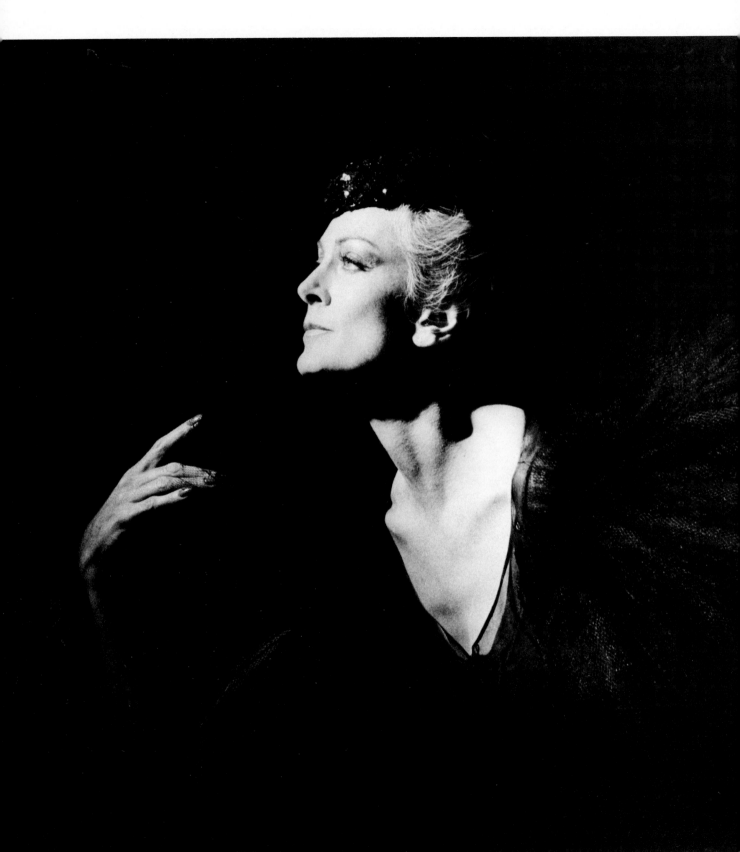

5

CHANGE OF LIFE

SOME PEOPLE CALL IT "MEN-opause," but that's a misnomer. Menopause may be the most traumatic, but it is only one of a series of changes that begin to take place in a woman's body between the ages of forty-five and fifty-five. Collectively, they are known as the *climacteric.* The word is derived from the Greek *klimakter,* which literally means rung of a ladder. I find the image pleasing, because I like to think that at this critical point in our lives we are on a ladder and can either climb up or go down. The choice is ours. It indicates that we women do have choices, some control over our destinies, even at the important turning points.

To me, up is always better when on the ladder of life. Down is too often a descent into a depression foisted upon us by the attitudes of

Anticipate every phase of life. Fear is a woman's worst enemy. (*Bill Betterson*)

others. Sociologists have reported that change of life is almost never a problem for women in cultures in which there is a great respect for age. It is only in youth-addicted societies that it may become nearly insupportable.

Despite a lingering worship of youth, the signs are good for a lessening of the psychological impact of the climacteric in our country. We American women are no longer finding our identities only through our men and our children. As our value stops being measured by our ability to bear children, the end of that ability should stop being a great problem.

Recently, looking through the newspaper for the announcement of the marriage of a friend's daughter, I was struck by how much more than wives and mothers many of us have already become. Almost all of the brides were working in doctoral programs, completing advanced professional degrees, or already had careers. More significantly, most of their mothers also had responsible positions outside the home. Our collective status seemed no longer to be achieved in the maternity ward and terminated at menopause. Because our sense of self-worth can come from so many sources other than being wives and mothers, chances are the majority of us will be able to join the many women who experience change of life with no serious side effects.

Before examining the conditions that occur during the climacteric and what can be done to help, there is one point I would like to make as strongly as I possibly can. The change is a natural part of a woman's life. It is not a disease or an illness. Generally, only when it does *not* occur is there the possibility of a serious medical condition.

MENOPAUSE

Menopause is actually the second great physiological change in a woman. The first is puberty, which marks the beginning of our ability to bear children, just as menopause is the end of it. That is all it is—the end of our reproductive powers. It is not the end of our value as individuals. It is certainly not the end of our sex lives. We are still capable of orgasm and of very rich and rewarding sensual experiences. In fact, some women enjoy sex more after menopause simply because there is no longer any danger of conception.

There are many theories as to why menopause begins at different ages in different women, but there are exceptions to all of them. It is widely believed that women who enter puberty early will reach the menopause late and vice versa. I'm an exception to that theory. As I've already said, I was a late bloomer, and I've yet to enter menopause. Other theories are that a woman who has never had a child will generally have an early menopause; that poor women reach menopause before rich women; that thin women have a later menopause than fat ones;

and that women of color have earlier menopause than those with fair skin.

Heredity may determine when one has one's menopause. I think, however, that the rich-poor and fat-thin theories merit an additional observation. Obviously, the woman who eats a balanced diet with sound nutritional values and who has the time to exercise regularly will be in good health and shape. It may well be that this contributes to a prolongation of her fertile period as well as an easier passage through the climacteric when it does arrive. Several of the gynecologists I've consulted agree that this is a very strong possibility.

Irregular menstrual bleeding is generally the first signal of the beginning of menopause. The period may be late; sometimes a whole month can be missed. It can be heavy one month and light the next, no more than a few drops. Although some women may abruptly stop menstruating, for most of us it happens gradually and can take anywhere from several months to two years. Twelve months after the last period, a woman is generally no longer fertile. However, because there is a danger of miscalculation and our bodies sometimes do act in mysterious ways, many gynecologists suggest that we continue to use contraception for twelve months to two years after we appear to have passed the menopause. This is especially true for women under fifty. Even if we are premenopausal, we should stop using the pill by the time we reach forty-two because of potentially dangerous side effects and the possibility of misleading bleeding even after the onset of the climacteric.

SOME PHYSIOLOGICAL CHANGES. Aside from the loss of fertility, the most acute physiological change that we experience during the climacteric is a drastic drop in the ovarian production of the female hormones, progesterone and especially estrogen. Many of the accompanying effects of menopause can be traced to this reduction. However, we cannot discount the psychological contribution to such symptoms as palpitations, depression, digestive problems, overweight, and breathlessness. We are at a traumatic and crucial point in our lives. If those we love do not react with tenderness and understanding, we can turn in upon ourselves.

I cannot emphasize strongly enough that only 10 percent of us suffer from severe symptoms of any kind, and even those of us who do are still basically healthy. They are symptoms of the climacteric and, I repeat, that is not a disease. The discomforts are generally of short duration, and most of us are strong enough to cope with them, just as we did with the discomforts of the onset of early puberty.

For the majority, the loss of ovarian estrogen does not present a large problem. The body compensates by producing large amounts of the male hormone androgen, which is converted into estrogen. Only in the most extreme cases should estrogen-replacement therapy be contemplated, and then only in small doses for the shortest possible time. Whether estrogen is taken in the form of pills or externally applied creams, the growing evidence of a link between its use and the development of uterine and breast cancers is too great to ignore.

HOT FLASHES. Hot flashes are among the most common symptoms of the climacteric. They may begin before the periods stop and continue for two or more years after menopause. The flash usually starts with a hot sensation in the chest and spreads up to the neck and head, bringing an uncomfortable blush to the face. Sometimes it starts in the feet and spreads, bringing a distinct tingling to other parts of the body. At their worst, they can awaken one in the middle of the night with a cold sweat.

Hot flashes can last from a few seconds up to several minutes. They can occur many times during a day or infrequently over a longer period of time. Unless you are one of that small minority who find the flashes utterly unendura-ble, the temptation of estrogen therapy must be avoided. There are safer alternatives. Some women have found vitamin E and ginseng-extract supplements helpful. If the flashes occur during periods of great tension or stress, tranquilizers may alleviate the symptoms. Many gynecologists prescribe either Clomiphene or Norethindrone for severe cases. Only when all else fails should we consider estrogen.

ITCHING AND DRYNESS. During the climacteric, the drop in female hormones can cause itching in many parts of the body, particularly in the vagina. There are many creams and ointments that a physician can prescribe to alleviate the problem. Again, estrogen creams are the last resort and, if used at all, should be used very sparingly for a carefully proscribed length of time.

Thinning of the vaginal lining, shrinkage, and dryness are also not uncommon symptoms. They can make intercourse difficult, but in most cases the use of a lubricating jelly before sex will eliminate the difficulties.

PREMENSTRUAL SYNDROME. The premenstrual symptoms that many women experience during the second half of the menstrual cycle—tenderness in the breasts, dysmenorrhea, weight gain, headaches, bloating, edginess—are often experienced by women in the years just before the menopause. It has nothing to do with the estrogen level but is symptomatic of a change in the progesterone balance. The condition will disappear after menopause; in the meantime, if one cannot cope, progesterone therapy in small doses will relieve the problem. Although progesterone has none of the dangerous potential of estrogen, it is still a hormone and should be used with extreme care and only under the supervision of a doctor.

MENOPAUSAL SYNDROME. What some physicians persist in calling the "menopausal syndrome" is really a catchall for most of the symptoms a woman may complain of as she approaches menopause. These include palpitations, headaches, breathlessness, flatulence, dizzy spells, ennui, insomnia, constipation or diarrhea, and listlessness. Not all are experienced by every woman (some women never suffer from any of them), and there is no rhythm or predictability about which will occur when. The truth is that nobody has ever proved that these symptoms are directly related to menopause at all. As a matter of fact, if we think back on all of our experiences during menstrual cycles since puberty, most of us will find that we have suffered from one or another of these complaints at some point during our adult lives. It is only natural that we be conscious of every change in balance as we go through the climacteric, but we mustn't allow ourselves to become unduly alarmed. They are neither serious nor lasting and will pass in a relatively short time.

CHANGE OF LIFE AND CHANGE OF PROPORTIONS. Change of life does not cause weight gain. If we do experience an increase in weight, it can be attributed to a natural slowing down that comes to all of us as we get older. We are taking in the same amount of food but using less energy and burning up fewer calories. The easy solution to the problem is to watch our diets and to exercise.

Even if we do not gain weight as we approach the end of the climacteric, there may be a discernible change in our dimensions. The breasts may sag, and there may be a thickening in the waist, thighs, and upper arms. Our bottoms may obey the rules of gravity and start sinking toward the ground. Some women have themselves reshaped surgically or try hormone therapy. I think those are the courts of last appeal. What we have to do is prime those muscles, get them working again—in short, it seems to me that exercise is the safest and sanest way to get rid of the problems.

AFTER MENOPAUSE

According to my own admittedly very personal timetable, middle age does not begin until after the climacteric. As long as we are capable of conceiving, we are young. Some of us have half a lifetime ahead of us, and even by conservative estimates we can look forward to one-third. These can be wonderful, constructive, fulfilling years, but only if we take care of ourselves. Our health is the key to our happiness and our beauty. With very few exceptions, the illnesses that may befall us at this time are common to both sexes and have nothing to do with so-called female complaints. Many can be avoided or at least ameliorated by proper diet and sufficient exercise. These are the keys to health and longevity, and most women of our age seem to pay more attention to them than do our male contemporaries. This may well be a large contributing factor to our statistically longer life expectancy.

Although cancer strikes both sexes in equal numbers, there are those specific to women. We are most susceptible in middle age and must be constantly on the lookout for symptoms.

BREAST CANCER. Whether or not changes in the estrogen level have any connection with breast cancer is still under investigation, but it does strike women most often immediately before, during, and just after the climacteric (ages forty to sixty). Monthly self-examination is vital. If there is any change or a lump develops, a physician must be consulted immediately. The chances are it will not be cancer—but if it is, early detection can save a life.

CERVICAL CANCER. Next to breast cancer, cervical cancer is the most dangerous female cancer. Fifty percent of the cases are fatal. As in all cancers, the difference between life and death is early detection. An annual Pap test is essential for every woman until she reaches the age of sixty-five.

UTERINE CANCER. Cancer of the lining of the uterus is one of the most common of the female reproductive-tract cancers. It usually afflicts women over fifty. As in cervical cancer, the first sign is generally abnormal bleeding during menstruation, between periods, or after menopause. It seems most common in women who have never been pregnant, or are obese, or have diabetes. The Pap test will usually not detect it, but a minisuction or lavaging procedure will usually enable the physician to obtain uterine cells for analysis. These tests can be performed in a physician's office, and women in any of the above high-risk categories should have them routinely.

OVARIAN TUMORS. Most ovarian tumors are benign, but any abnormal growth has to be investigated. For this reason, all of us must continue to have regular gynecologic examinations even after the climacteric.

RHEUMATOID ARTHRITIS AND OSTEOPOROSIS. These are two diseases to which middle-aged women are more susceptible than men or women in any other group. Although not fatal, they are both debilitating and can cause alterations in our routines.

Arthritis is actually a range of diseases causing redness, painful swelling, and in some cases permanent damage to the joints. Rheumatoid arthritis usually begins in middle age and afflicts three times as many women as it does men. In most cases, it initially appears in the first joints of the fingers, but it can show up in any joints. It is a chronic condition, but it can be controlled. What happens is an overproduction of tissue around the joints, which leads to inflammation, swelling, and ultimately degeneration of the joints as well as the tendons, cartilage, and ligaments connected to them.

Although there is a range of drugs that can be prescribed, plain aspirin is the most effective in a majority of cases. Applications of heat are also helpful. The arthritic person should have regular rest periods each day, but the rest should be accompanied by a program of exercises designed to strengthen the muscles around the affected joints.

Osteoporosis seems to be the one disease that has a direct relationship to the reduction of estrogen in our bodies after the climacteric. Pockets form inside the bones, making them brittle and susceptible to fracture even from a seemingly insignificant fall or bruise.

There is no treatment that will strengthen the bones, but regular exercise will build the muscles around them, providing additional protection, and will also help to metabolize calcium, thus helping to prevent greater deterioration. Every woman of our age should take approximately 1,000 milligrams of calcium daily. It is available in dairy products. Taking it orally in the form of pill or capsule does not help this condition. It must come from foodstuffs. Vitamin D–fortified low-fat milk is one of the best sources. The milk is rich in calcium, and vitamin D promotes its absorption.

I have already spoken of the danger of injections or oral supplements of pure estrogen. It will lessen the chance of osteoporosis, but there is the link to cancer that must be considered. Gynecologic experts have come up with a solution—a formula that combines estrogen with progesterone and thus far seems to have eliminated the danger of cancer.

This substance would appear to be a true wonder for those of us experiencing the climacteric or having passed it. It all but eliminates hot flashes. It inhibits osteoporosis. It increases vaginal lubrication while reducing shrinkage. It stimulates the secretions of the sebaceous glands, which keeps our skin from drying. It prevents our hair from thinning.

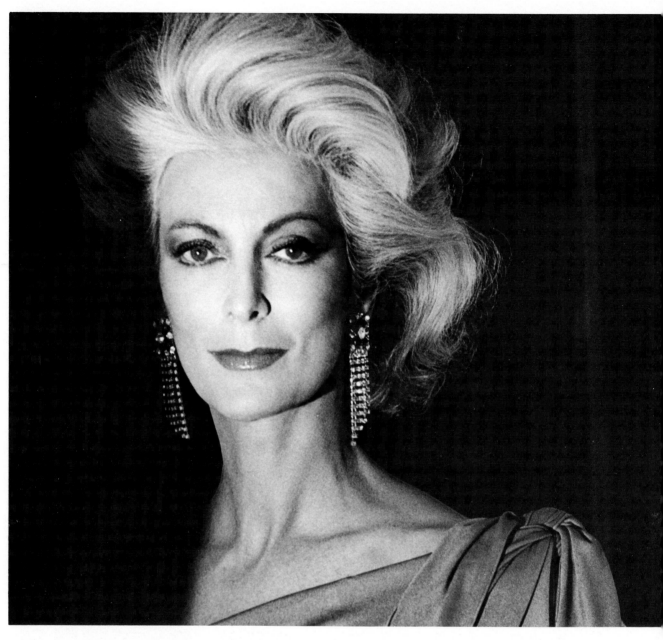

A close-up taken as recently as November 1984. *(David King)*

It sounds as if the estrogen-progesterone formula is the miracle for which we've all been waiting, but this is not always the case. Each of us is different, and there are dangers in it for some women. Discuss all of the implications, pro and con, with your gynecologist. If he or she has any reservations, don't try it. It is possible that your doctor will have an alternative. Osteoporosis has become an important research field. By the time you read this, there may be some new and remarkable breakthrough that will eliminate the danger of the disease and without possible perilous side effects.

In middle age, beauty is health, and that makes the physician the greatest beauty expert in the world. How well we look is governed by how well our internal organs are functioning. Before attempting any radical change in our normal regimens, we should consult a doctor so that we are aware of how it may affect our overall well-being.

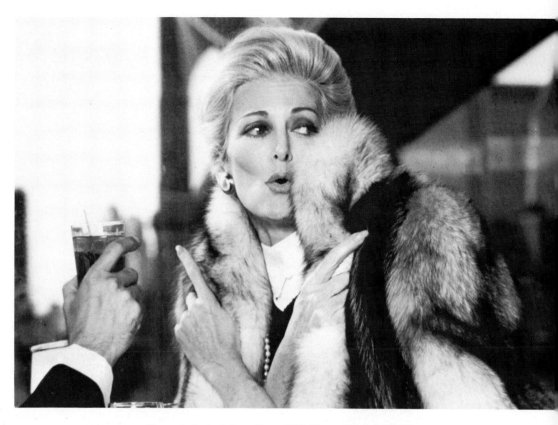

Recent shots taken for a TV client. (*Henry Wolf*)

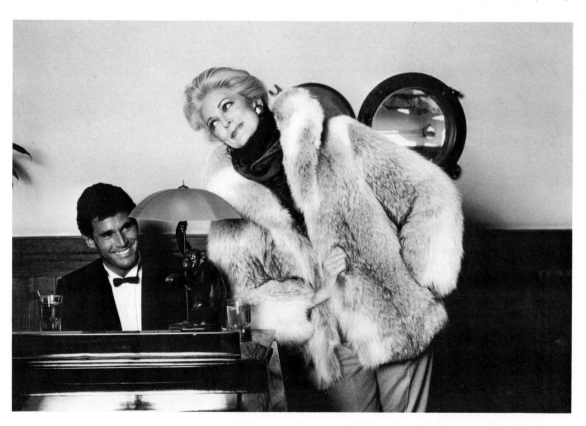

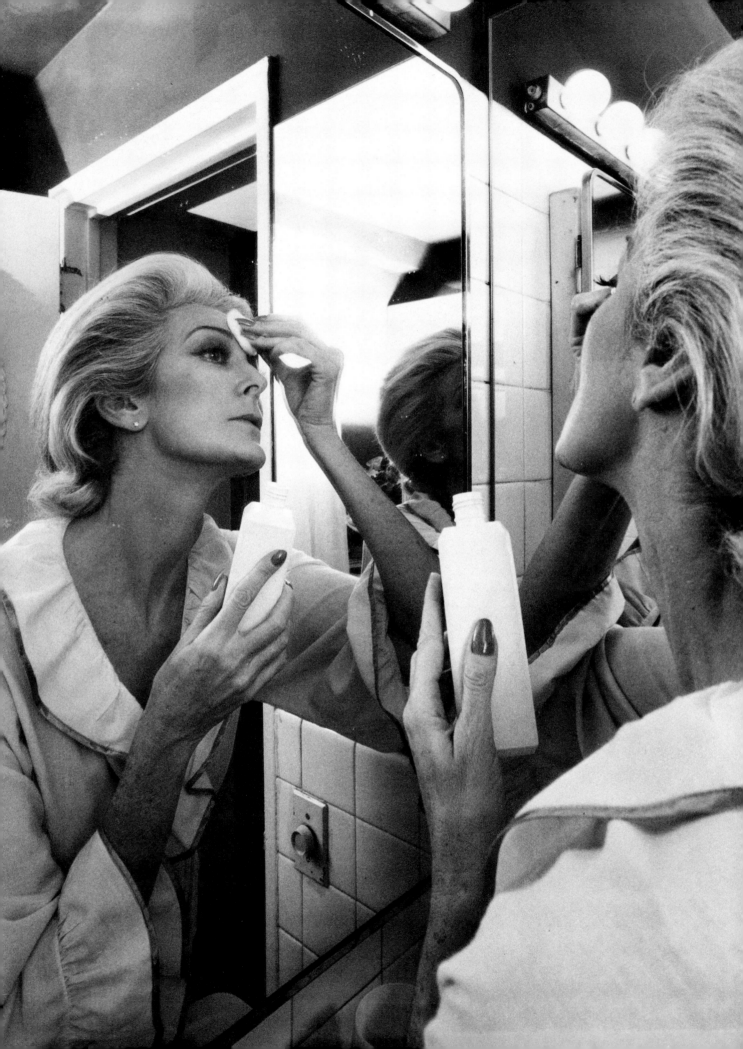

6

COSMETICS

MERICAN MEN AND
women spend upwards of $10 billion a year on
cosmetics. Yes, men are almost as heavily into
the stuff as we are, so don't let any of them try
to put you down for buying that extra lipstick.
Just take a look at the cosmetics section of your
favorite department store. You'll find counters
cluttered with moisturizers, toners, astringents,
scents, and bronzers made specifically for the
male of the species, and they're doing a brisk
business, with the lads being offered overnight
cases, jackets, toiletries kits, and umbrellas as
inducements to buy, buy, buy. Every leading
cosmetics company has a special male line, and
if you look at the lists of ingredients, you'll find
they are putting on their faces exactly what we

I've learned to take the time to pamper myself.

are putting on ours. There are best-selling
beauty books written especially for men. Why
not? I think it's wonderful that they are finally
liberated enough to confess they have the same
fears, insecurities, vanities, and needs we have.

Even though cosmetics are regulated by the
FDA, which defines them as articles which may
be "rubbed, poured, sprinkled, or sprayed on,
introduced into, or otherwise applied to the
human body for cleansing, beautifying, pro-
moting attractiveness, or altering the appearance without affecting the body's structure or
functions."

For the public, probably the most significant
difference between a drug and a cosmetic is that
a drug must be proven safe and effective before
it is put on the market. Although the FDA can
have a cosmetic removed from the market if it
actually proves unsafe, they have no control

over the claims made for it. Claims can be as extravagant as a manufacturer chooses to make them, but we don't have to believe them. What we choose to believe is subject to our hopes and dreams, which cannot be regulated by the government.

Fortunately, manufacturers are required to list the ingredients in their products, and no matter what the brand name, the ingredients are basically the same, with one or two minor additives. If you have an allergic reaction to any product, obviously you should stop using it. Then check the ingredients listed on the label with your physician to learn what you are reacting badly to, so you can avoid it in other products.

Most cosmetic products are harmless, but they offer no magic beyond what you choose to believe. Whatever help they give comes from artful application and consistent use as part of a beauty regimen. The one good reason for using well-known and expensive brands is that the larger companies have good laboratory facilities for checking safety. It is good business for them not to put out a dangerous product they will subsequently have to withdraw if the FDA finds it unsafe.

What I want to say has been summed up in a pamphlet, *Aging Skin,* put out by the Department of Health Education of the American Medical Association.

There are no "miracle cosmetics," but use of cosmetics can minimize some effects of the aging process and delay others. The vast majority of cosmetic preparations in the United States are safe and can be used with confidence. Ingredients that have caused undesirable reactions are largely omitted from today's preparations. The problems that do arise are generally a result of misleading terminology and exaggerated claims used in some advertising materials.

For example, beware of advertisements that promise (directly or indirectly) that a certain cream will remove wrinkles or restore youthful beauty. *There is no cream, no matter how expensive, that will safely and effectively remove or prevent wrinkles.* Products containing ingredients such as royal jelly, placental extract, tur-

tle oil, mink oil, natural proteins, polyunsaturates, or "secret formulas" are usually safe to use, but they have not been scientifically proven to rejuvenate aged skin. They are merely good cold creams or vanishing creams, sold at an exorbitant price, and are useful only as such. Most preparations do what any good emollient cream or lotion will do for the skin: they temporarily make fine surface lines less prominent, and they supply oil and moisture to combat dryness and roughness. They soften the skin by retarding evaporation of the water that reaches the outer horny layer from underlying tissue. Repeated use of a good quality cream may alleviate the dryness and scaling that add to the signs of aging skin.

Never shortchange a dream. If you have a product you believe in, keep on using it no matter what any self-appointed "expert" says. Part of how we look is mind over matter. When we think we look good, we generally do look better; and when we think we're looking our worst, we often do. There are women who gain confidence from using the best in the sense of the most expensive. If they can afford it, more power to them. That confidence is going to be as efficacious to their looks as any of the ingredients. But we must beware of the economics trap. Nothing ages us as quickly as financial problems. We mustn't let advertisements or claims coerce us into spending more than we can afford. The budget squeeze is going to add more worry lines than any surgeon or pharmaceutical product can ever erase.

With cosmetics, consistency is the secret of success. I have a daily beauty routine from which I never stray, no matter how tired or pressed for time I may be.

My day begins with a shower. Three times a week, I use the Buf-Puf on my face (see p. 177) and on those parts of my body that seem dry, concentrating on the feet, knees, backs of the arms, and elbows.

After showering, I spread on a thin layer of body lotion. I use a scented lotion because my body can tolerate it, but that's one of the tricky points. Whenever I've had an allergic reaction to a cosmetic, it's been to the added perfumes, so I think most people are safer with unscented products.

Next, I apply a healthy coat of moisturizer to my face and neck. Some of you may be thinking I've skipped a step. What about the astringent that's so often recommended for use before the moisturizer? I no longer use it. That's one of the things I stopped doing after my reappraisal in my forties. As I've gotten older, my skin has become too dry, and an astringent further depletes the lessened supply of natural sebaceous-gland secretions. With an oily skin, the astringent step should be part of the treatment, but the only time I use one is to dab it on for freshening when my skin feels tired during the day.

I let the moisturizer sink in while I prepare my breakfast. Part of my beauty routine is to drink a glass of hot water with the juice of a fresh lemon in it. I rub my elbows with the rind. The few drops of juice remaining, combined with the natural fruit oils in the rind, work wonders with the thin layer of skin in that area. After breakfast, I blot my face with a cotton pad and apply a second coat of moisturizer, very sparingly, so that it is absorbed quickly. If you have oily skin, skip this step completely. Your skin doesn't need additional moisture.

MAKEUP. If she chooses, a young woman can think of her unlined face as a blank canvas and use heavy, oily makeup to paint on whatever face she fancies. I think it's a terrible idea at any age, but youth does have that option. The older woman must forgo that approach. Her face is a piece of sculpture carved by time and experience. The color she applies must be muted and as delicately tinted as a watercolor. Any harshness only serves to emphasize the sculptural details she wants to soften.

In my forties, I started to spend a great deal less money on makeup. It was not that I was wearing much less, it was only that I eliminated all of the chichi, high-fashion frills. No glitter, much less gloss, no more rainbow of colors intended to accessorize my wardrobe at the expense of my face. Everything was brought down to the basics that were best for me at my age. After all, my features were my statement and my style; I refused to sacrifice them to "their" fashion of the year.

There are exceptions to every rule, but, generally speaking, there are a few cosmetic verities that should be observed by every woman over forty, because there is no exception to time passing.

- Less is more. Makeup will emphasize or de-emphasize, but it can never cover up.
- No earthy, muddy, brown colors. They drain natural color at a time when it is beginning to fade.
- No blues or yellows. The blue turns the skin ashen and the yellow makes it look sallow. This includes the secondary colors of orange, lavender, magenta, violet, green.
- A fresh, crisp mouth ranging from warm pink to pure red.
- No black lines around the eyes.
- No cake makeup. Use liquid and creamy foundations and blushers that aid in moisturizing.
- As little eye shadow as possible, and no definite fashion color. A shade of tan deeper than one's foundation, or gray, perhaps taupe on the dark-skinned woman.
- As little powder as possible. What powder we use should be extremely fine and very lightly misted over the face. Powder gets into fine lines and emphasizes them. None should be applied around the eyes or lips. Too much powder cakes and makes the skin look dry and flaky.

Before deciding on a makeup, it's an excellent idea to go to the mirror and take a good look at yourself without any makeup on and in the brightest daylight. Wear your eyeglasses or contacts if you need them. You want to see the sharpest possible image of your unadorned features. Nature does help illusion by weakening our vision at the point in our lives when we'd most like to blur the fine lines she's adding to our faces.

The eyes and mouth are the dominant areas for tonal emphasis. Now that you're in sharp focus, decide which is best. Always staying within the guidelines I've set down above, play up the best feature in your face. A good mouth deserves a bright, fresh color. Good eyes can take shadow and a more defined line. If it is a toss-up between the two, strike a cosmetic balance by either heightening or muting, depending on what you see.

After you've put on your makeup, take another good look in bright daylight. You'll soon know if your face is ready for street wear. If adjustments are called for, it's certainly worth taking the few minutes needed to make them. I'm not advocating tardiness for either a business or a social engagement. It's a question of arranging our old friend and enemy, time, for all contingencies.

Craig Gadson is one of the brightest young makeup artists around. He's been invaluable to me at sittings and fashion shows. Although still in his early twenties, Craig loves the challenge of working on mature women. He has come up with a makeup that will work for every woman no matter what her age, shape, or color. The application is constant, but there are certain tonal differences that depend on the shade of the skin.

For all women, the foundation should be sheer, translucent, slightly tinted but as close as possible to the natural shade of the skin. Powder should be used sparingly if at all. Even with an oily skin, it is often better to blot excess moisture and oil pockets with a tissue and let the natural glow shine through than it is to powder. Each woman must judge for herself, but generally the matte finish of powder emphasizes lines.

FAIR SKIN
 Lips: Pink to pure red, depending on how much attention is to be drawn to them.

Cheeks: Rose, peach, pink. Liquid rouge or blusher.
 Eyes: Dark gray liner. With blue or gray eyes, perhaps a charcoal brown to warm them up. Dark tan or taupe eye shadow.

OLIVE SKIN
 Lips: Pure tones of coral, red, or rose.
 Cheeks: Blusher of same color as lips.
 Eyes: Dark gray liner. Taupe shadow.

BLACK SKIN
 Lips: Bright red. The only skin type that might even go for mandarin orange.
 Cheeks: Dabs of her lipstick carefully blended in.
 Eyes: Black liner (it will turn a warm gray on her skin). Taupe or charcoal brown eye shadow, whichever is a tone darker than her skin.

A woman with a ruddy complexion should wear a clear, bright color on her lips and nothing on her cheeks. Her natural coloring provides all the tonal enhancement she needs. She should play it up if for no better reason than that she can't play it down without turning her face into an unsightly painted mask.

With few exceptions, women over forty should throw away their false eyelashes. They cast terrible shadows and only draw attention to the lines beginning to form around the eyes. The exceptions are women with very sparse lashes. To fill in, they should cut tiny clusters of false lashes from the band to apply to the thinned-out places, but it must be very delicately done and never the full band favored by the Hollywood glamour girls of the 1940s.

I dye my eyelashes. Not only does it save time but it's a far more natural look and eliminates the risk of unattractive beading. No matter what your coloring, I think your lashes should be black, because it gives both clarity and definition.

The key is simplification. With so many cosmetics on the market, you can get lost and confused, not know what to buy. Disregard the

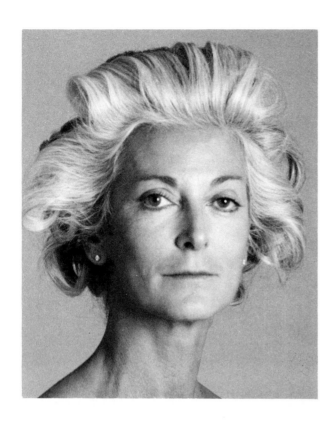

A cleansed and moisturized face ready for the application of make up.

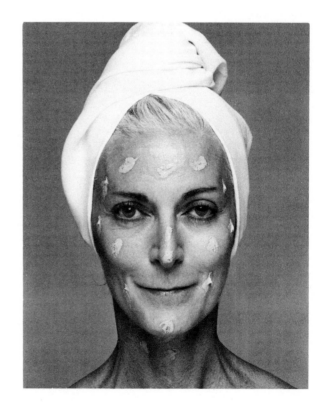

Apply daubs of foundation all over the face. With the balls of your fingers, spread it to within one-quarter inch of the hairline and down over the neck.

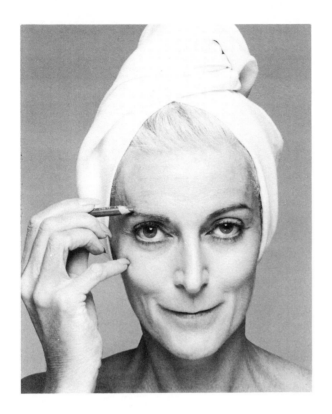

The eyebrow should neither be plucked too thin nor left bushy. The happy medium is the rule. Apply an eyebrow pencil with fine, feathery strokes. No harsh, unbroken lines.

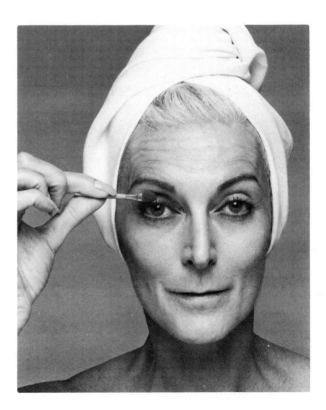

Apply shadow to the lower lid with an applicator. Remember, no glaring "designer" colors.

158

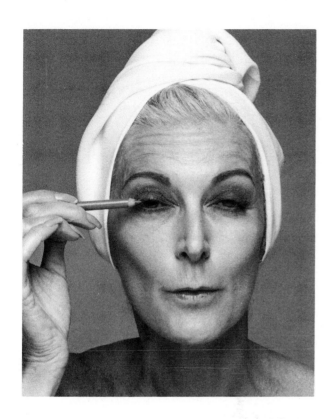

The eye-liner pencil is used above and as close to the lashes as possible. Select a gray or taupe shade. No black lines.

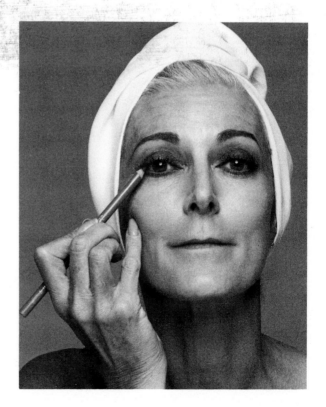

Apply a fine line just below the upper lashes using the same pencil.

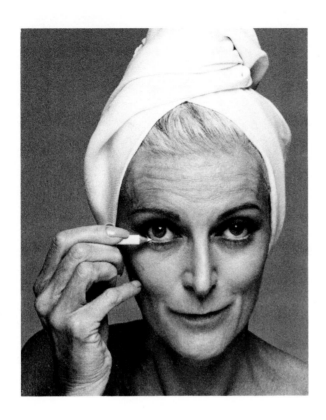

A white pencil can be used just above the lower lashes to make the eyes look larger, brighter, and clearer.

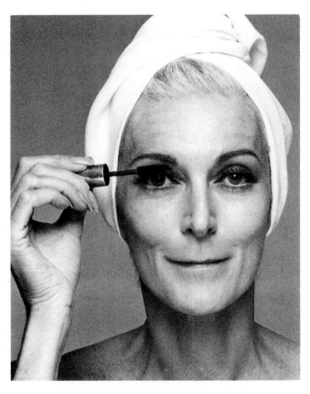

Apply mascara to the upper lashes. You may use a lash curler but, generally, it isn't necessary. These days, the applicators do a fine job of curling and even extending the lashes. Never use false lashes unless the real ones have fallen out.

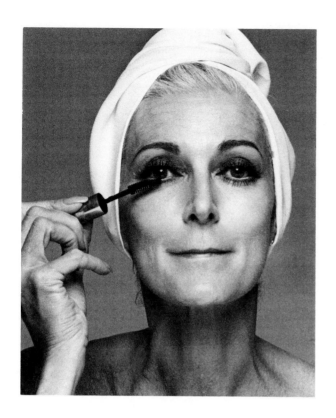

Delicately apply mascara to the lower lashes so that each one is done individually and there are no bubbles.

Using a lighter shade of your foundation or a translucent lightener (a shade lighter but never white), dot the places where there are creases or shadows on your face. Also place daubs on the upper lids just under the eyebrows. Delicately blend these spots in with the ball of your finger as if you were delicately rubbing out the shadows and creases. The blended in daubs on the upper lids will brighten your eyes and bring them out.

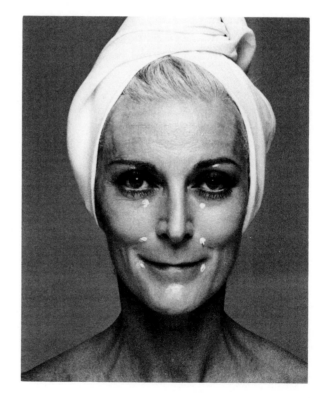

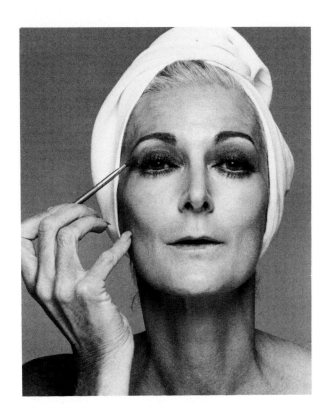

Blend a little rouge with your powder and apply it to the creases between the upper and lower lids. This will eradicate the harsh line between mascara and highlight and give the eyes a finished, natural look.

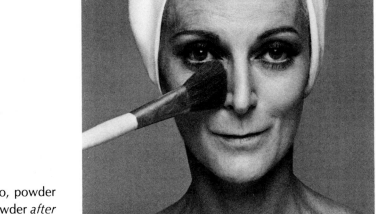

If you use a cream-based make up, as I do, powder now. If you use a water-based make up, powder *after* completing the contouring steps 13 through 17. Don't forget to powder the lips.

162

We are ready for contouring. The rule is if you use a cream-based foundation, you must use a cream-based blusher or rouge for contouring. If you use a water-based foundation, then it must be a water-based cosmetic for contouring. Let me repeat, it's cream on cream and water on water.

Study your face to be certain that you need contouring. If your jawline is firm, and you like your nose the way it is, *do not* contour. It's just adding more make up at a time when you really want to use less.

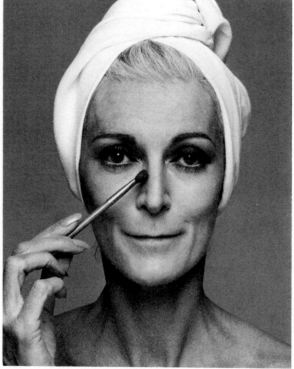

To contour the nose, thin your blusher down with powder and delicately apply it to the sides of your nose from eyes to just above the nostrils. We thin the blusher down so that there will be no unsightly dark and obviously made up patches on the face.

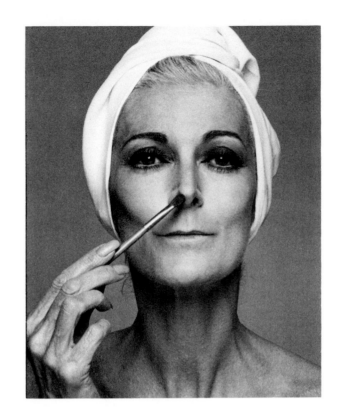

Contour the small dimples at the tip of the nose with the thinned-down blusher.

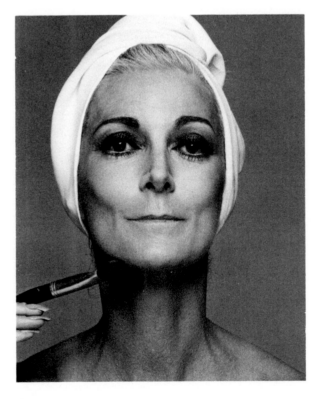

Use a brush to contour along the chin and jaw, then blend the thinned-down blusher down over the neck to get rid of any harsh lines and create a natural looking shadow.

164

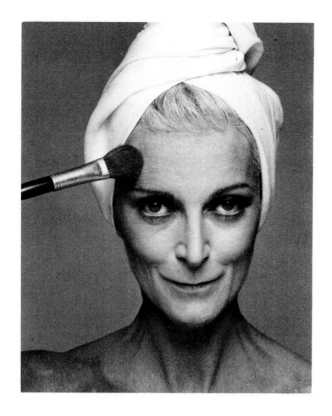

Deepen the temples with thinned-down blusher.

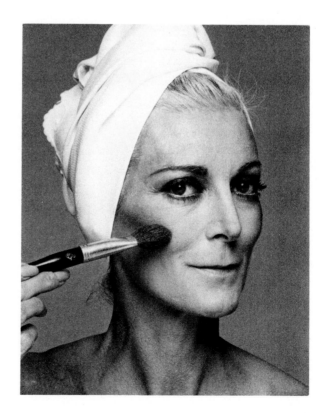

Apply the blusher to the plane of the cheek-bones. This is the only place on my face where I use the blusher in full intensity without any thinning down with powder.

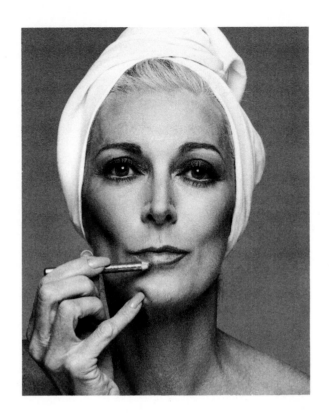

Outline the mouth with a pencil as close in tone to your lipstick as possible. This outline will contain the grease in the lipstick and prevent it from spreading into the fine lines around the mouth.

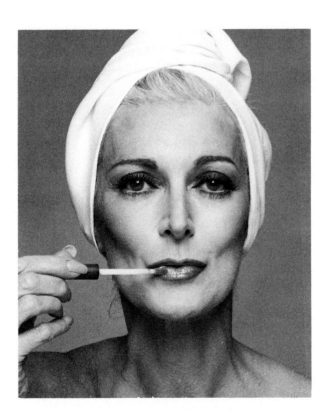

Fill in the mouth with lipstick or gloss.

166

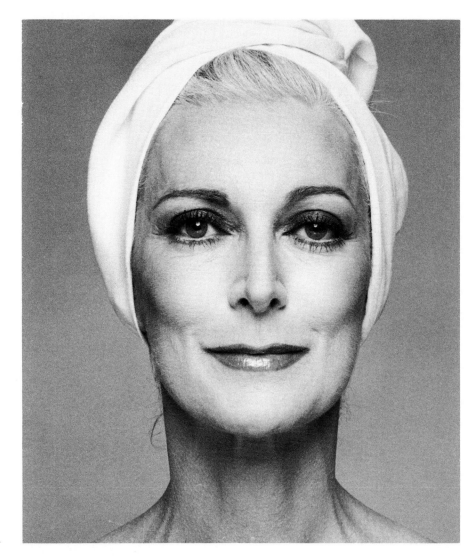

The completed make up.

fleeting and the trendy. Come down to a narrow range, for within it, you will be your most beautiful. Don't strive for the impossible. Respect yourself, and let your own magnificence shine through an understated face. I know it takes courage to accept what is inside rather than superimposing fashion's false image, but to survive intact to our age took an abundance of courage, so the courage is there—let's use it!

In the evening, I sometimes smear the smallest dabs of Vaseline on my lips, across the tops of my cheekbones, under my eyes, and on the lids. This adds a dewy "wet" look that I find both very attractive and youthful. It casts a lovely glow on the face in the artificial and dimmer evening light. Again, I emphasize, use the tiniest amount and so well spread that it disappears as Vaseline and remains as only the most subtle gleam on the skin.

If I'm wearing a particularly spectacular evening dress, I might add a little glitter to my eyes and a gloss to my lips. These are rare and special occasions when the dress itself is a costume and allows for a certain artificial theatricality in the makeup. Usually, I just heighten my normal makeup. The eye shadow and lips are a tone darker. The brows and lashes are accentuated. But nothing is overdone.

If I have a date in the evening, the ideal is to remove all makeup and start anew, but sometimes I don't have the time. In that case, I blot my nose, around my eyes, and brow with a cotton pad soaked in astringent. I then apply a light coat of a cream-based foundation, because it has a moisturizer, which my skin needs by this time of day. For blending in with the makeup already on my face, a shade slightly lighter than the original works best.

Before going to bed, I run a tub with some bath oil in the water. While it is filling, I use a heavy cold cream or mineral oil to remove every bit of my makeup. After I've wiped it off, I do a light half-creaming, removing it with a washcloth but leaving a slight film on my face when I get into the tub. By the time I've finished my bath, the combination of steam and cream has given a soft and fresh feeling to my skin.

I pierce a vitamin E capsule with a pin and remove a little of the oil, which I pat under and around my eyes. Before you try this, be sure you're not allergic to vitamin E. If you are, any eye cream that works for you will do as well to relax and feed this very dry area of the face.

My last step before going to bed is to apply a moisturizer or night cream. Cocoa butter or a light coat of mineral oil will do as well as any of the more expensive products. The important thing is, whether or not you sleep in a nightie, nobody should go to bed wearing nothing on the face.

NAILS. No more talons dripping blood! Our hands are aging along with the rest of us, and long, brightly colored nails only call attention to them. I keep my nails at medium length and polished with a neutral color. I've already given some diet suggestions that will help keep nails in good condition. Always wear rubber gloves when washing dishes or clothes or anything else except your hands and body. Water can make the nails brittle. Exercise your fingers every day. The simple act of typing or knitting will do the trick. Exercise strengthens the nails. When all else fails, you can resort to false nails. Better still, there are nail salons that specialize in building, extending, and sculpting. Brittle, broken, ugly nails can be transformed into things of beauty in just one sitting. The service may be a little expensive, but it is worth it and lasts quite a long time.

HAIR. There are excellent shampoos and conditioners on the market for every conceivable type of hair. Most of us know what works best for our hair. If there is any doubt, ask your favorite hairdresser for advice. The person who has worked on your hair successfully knows better than anybody else what it needs to keep it clean and healthy.

I wash my hair in the shower every other day,

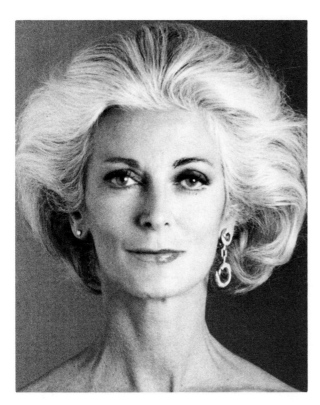

The right side of my face is made up for daytime and the left for evening. The difference is not a pronounced cosmetic alteration. It is simply a change in tone.

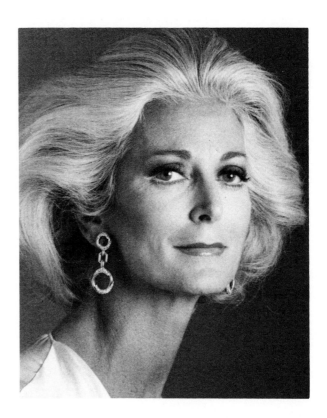

Ready to go out for the evening. Just a little more, but still a good deal less.

using an unscented shampoo. Cream rinses simply don't work for me—they make my hair too soft to hold a set. When I notice split ends, I use a protein conditioner, but only on the ends. This treatment works for me, but it's an individual thing and may not work for you. I have friends who do a full protein conditioning at least once a week. After years of living with their hair, they have discovered that it needs conditioning. It is right for them. Whatever keeps your hair lustrous, manageable, free of excess oil, and clean is right for you.

The two greatest hair problems for the older woman are thinning and graying. As we get older, we all start to lose some hair on our heads and to grow it in other, less appropriate places. Electrolysis, bleaches, waxing, and depilatories help to get rid of unwanted body and facial hair. To replace lost hair on the scalp, there are safe and easy transplants. Recently, doctors have been experimenting with estrogen drops applied directly to the scalp, which have proven safe and helpful in many cases. Good wigs are available in every conceivable shape, style, and color. If you can accustom yourself to wearing one, it saves a great deal of time and money at the beauty salon.

Styling can also be a great deceiver. I have this image of possessing a great mane of hair. Actually, my hair is straight and very thin. The appearance of thickness is very simple to create. After my shampoo, I give my hair a rinse with one tablespoon of vinegar mixed in a glass of water. It cuts the oil and makes my hair very dry and filled with electricity. I set it in very thick rolls. When I comb it out, it practically stands on end. All I have to do is lightly brush it back, and there is the illusion of enormous quantities of hair.

THE QUICK HAIR SET. I set my hair very quickly, and it works every single time. It needn't be after a vinegar rinse or a shampoo. I can do it between washings. The only impor-

tant note is to make certain that my hair is absolutely dry before I set it.

This set gives my hair body so that it doesn't simply hang down in a lifeless and lank fashion. The first few times, it helps to have a rear-view mirror. When you get the knack, you can do it by feel.

1. Starting at the front and center of forehead, comb up a healthy handful of hair about 3 inches wide. Apply some hair spray and over your finger roll it back away from the face into a fat sausage curl. Clip it in place.
2. Repeat this step three or four times until you reach the center of the scalp. Remember to spray each time before forming the curl and that all curls are rolled away from the face.
3. Using less hair, form smaller curls on both sides of the face. Clip each in place as you finish it. Don't forget the hair spray before forming the curls. Do this until all of your hair is curled except that mane which hangs down behind the center curls.
4. Repeat the small curls at the back of the head until all of your hair is curled.

After you've finished making your curls, give one final spray all over the head. When spray is dry to the touch, remove the clips. You don't have to wait. Comb out your hair teasing it up and away from your face.

On the subject of style, I think all of my contemporaries should wear their hair short and away from the face and shoulders. It can be either full or close to the skull, depending on individual preference. The important thing is that it must not hang down in anything resembling a long bob. If you love your long hair, wear it in a French twist or high bun. The sags and lines in our faces are the result of a combination of weakening muscles and gravity's pull. Hair that drapes down and rests on the shoulders also pulls our faces down and adds to the overall look of drooping fatigue. In everything we do with our faces and hair, we want to be high, light, airy. Sweep that hair up and away,

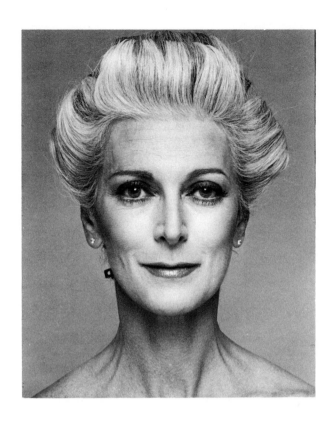

Front view of the fully curled head.

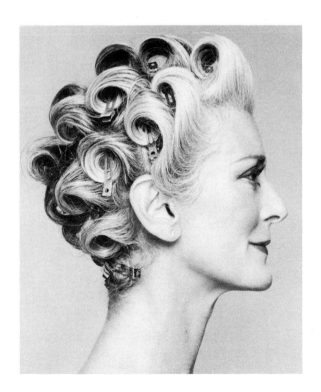

Profile view of the curled head.

171

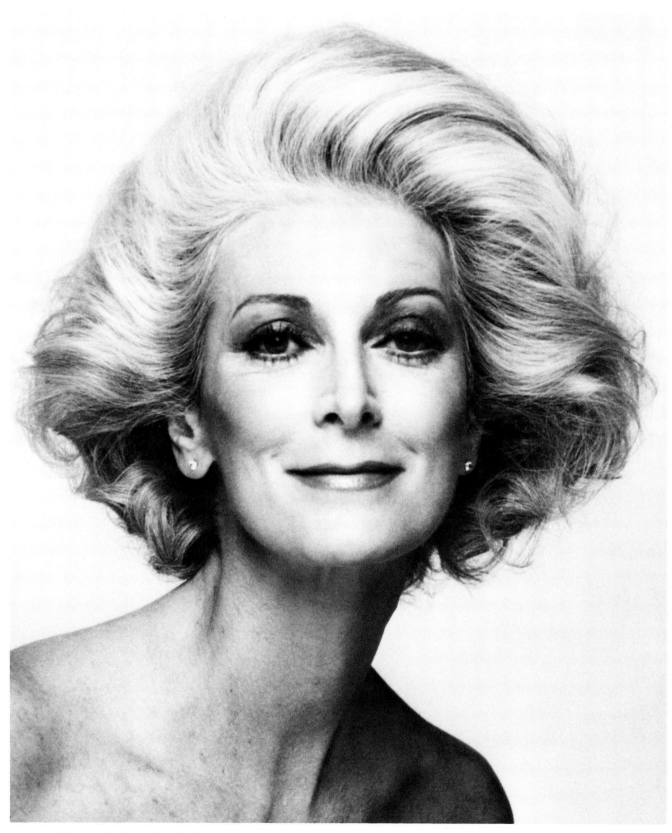

The combed out, finished set.

and the lines will seem to be swept up and away.

Gray hair is not actually a sign of aging. It is hereditary. I started to get gray in my early twenties, but I know women of sixty and older with naturally dark hair. Graying occurs when the pigment cells in the hair roots stop producing color. This usually starts to happen as we get older, although it is not necessarily the case.

Obviously, I like gray hair. I think any lighter shade of hair is much more becoming and youthful-looking on an older woman. It is nature's balance, lightening our hair as the pigment in our skin also begins to pale.

To accentuate my gray hair, I have the remaining dark hair highlighted by a process called frosting at Eva of New York. Frosting lightens the darker hair, thereby softening the contrast between dark and light hair. Eva has been gilding this lily for many years and was my main support when I went gray despite my husband's opposition.

For a woman with naturally dark hair, I suggest lightening the hair around the face. If she is going gray and doesn't like it, streaking the gray areas with a tone lighter than her natural hair is very becoming. Blondes should avoid brass and gold—they turn the skin sallow. Beige and ash tones are most becoming. For the gray-haired woman, lavender and blue rinses are disastrous because they age the skin and wash out what natural color she has.

The secret of beauty is naturalness, lightness, and balance. Hair should never be jarringly dark. Everything on the face and around it should blend to create a harmonious whole. Nothing should be out of tune or artificial. Too many women of my age use dyes and cosmetics as a way to "make up" for lost time instead of a way to keep up with the good times that are still coming.

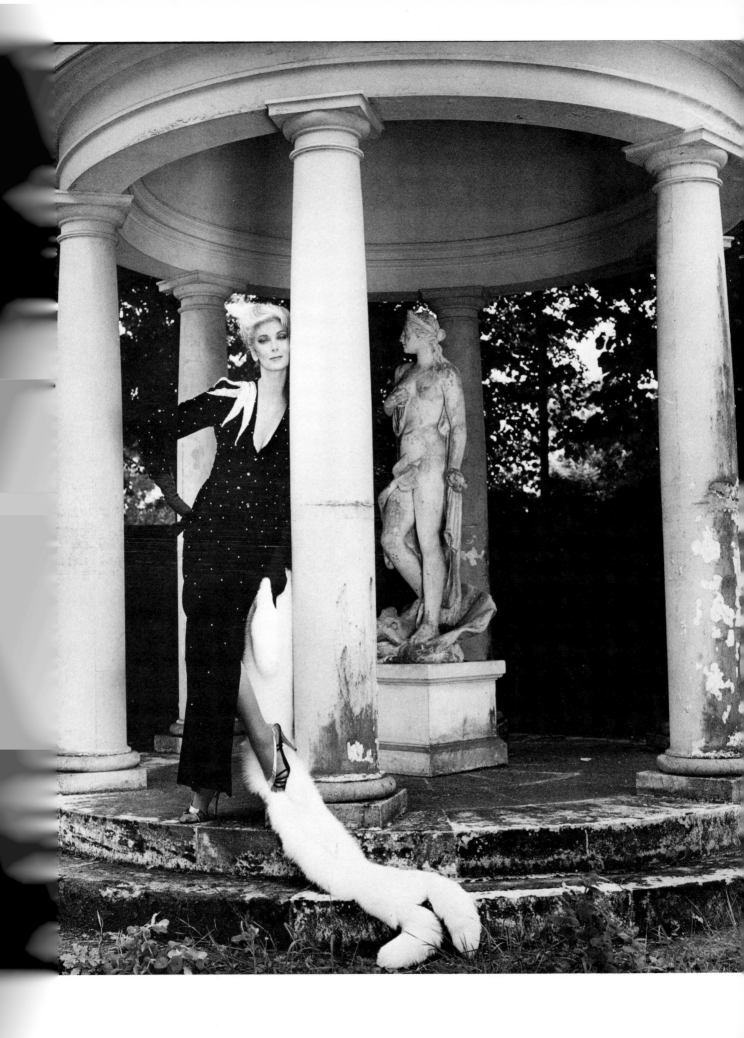

7

NEW FACES

THE EUPHEMISM IS, "HAVE you had a few nips and tucks?"

You'd be surprised at the number of people, including total strangers, who ask me that question. At the moment I'm writing this book, the answer is no, but by the time you read it—who knows? The query only indicates that the subject of plastic surgery is on most people's minds once they reach a certain age.

I have sought medical help for every physical problem I've ever had, and I see no reason to draw the line when the problem becomes my face. That face has already been helped by medicine. Had I not had my nose and teeth straightened in my adolescence, it would certainly not be the face you see now. I've also had some silicone implants above my lips (but more about

that presently). I don't know if any of these things would have been done had I been in another line of business. Certainly none was an effort to hold back time; they were done to lengthen a career. If photographs should show it's necessary, I'll have blepharoplasty (the technical name for an eye job) or even rhytidectomy (a face-lift).

With over 60 percent of the women in the work force, career has got to be one of the strongest motivations for seeking medical help with our appearances. It is a sad but true commentary on those in power, but women in the marketplace are often judged as much by their looks as by their abilities. Although they are at opposite ends of the feminine political spectrum, I've never seen either Gloria Steinem or Phyllis Schlafly display anything but shiningly well-groomed countenances in their public appearances. Our looks help us to make our points, no matter what those points may be.

Another photograph for French *Vogue*. (*Norman Parkinson*)

Anything that helps us to feel better is permissible, but when it comes to something as drastic as a face-lift, we should be sure we're not using the plastic surgeon as a substitute for a family counselor, psychoanalyst, divorce lawyer, or Ann Landers. He can lift the spirits as well as the face, but, as I've said, we remain the same women underneath. As potential patients, we can expect him to deal only with the physiognomy; the psyche is our own problem.

Before deciding to tamper with the face, an objective appraisal of it is in order. It is undoubtedly a good face that you've worn with dignity and pride for a long time. If there was anything drastically wrong, you would have done something about it a long time ago, just as I did with my nose and teeth. Now it is getting a little tired, perhaps even a little boring—after all, you have been looking at it every day of your life. The skin has lost some of its color and is noticeably drier. When you press the fleshy part with a finger, it doesn't spring back into place with the alacrity of youth. There are problems, but let's see if we've exhausted all of the many less troublesome solutions before resorting to the ultimate one. The lift is the court of last appeal, and it is an expensive, often painful appeal that is not always completely successful.

If the condition of the skin is the disturbing element, there are many simple ways of improving its quality without having to submit to therapeutics. Even if you should opt for a lift or any of the other medical treatments we will be discussing presently, these are things you should pay attention to as a matter of routine.

1. Get enough rest. Fatigue shows in the pallor and texture of the skin. We all know approximately how much rest we need in order to function at our best, and we must get it. The occasional sleepless night is no cause for alarm, but insomnia is a serious disease. See a doctor about it. A mild sedative or tranquilizer may be all that is necessary. In extreme cases, a sleep clinic is recommended because the sleep habits should be modified. More than the skin, one's entire physical well-being is at risk from want of adequate rest.

2. Follow the nutritional suggestions on page 143.

3. Never drop below 1,200 to 1,400 calories a day.

4. Follow the premakeup and postmakeup regimens outlined on pages 154–155, 156, 168.

5. Read the labels on all products that touch the face. The fewer chemical additives, the better they are.

6. Use as little soap as possible. A creamy cleansing agent with emollient properties is the best alternative. Most commercial soaps dry out the skin.

7. Stay out of the sun. How often that's been said, but it's like a voice in the wind. Women refuse to listen. No sunscreen or -block is 100 percent safe. Sun is the single most aging and destructive factor to the skin, and that includes the skin on any exposed part of the body. This sun worship is a throwback to the depression of the 1930s, when a tan indicated one was wealthy enough to afford a vacation. Why not let the lack of tan indicate that you are secure enough not to need this deleterious symbol?

EPIDERMABRASION. All of the lesser woes to which our flesh is heir are displayed in the epidermis: blackheads, whiteheads, blemishes, spots, blisters, and flaking. The epidermis is not one layer of skin but many layers of cells. Although you may not know it, we are constantly shedding our skins. New cells are being born in the lowest layer of the epidermis at this very moment. As they grow older, they will be pushed toward the surface by more new cells being generated beneath them. These old cells die on the surface and deaden the look of the skin with their thin, dull, dry, scaly, ashen appearance. Eventually, they flake or are washed off, carrying with them dirt, oily wastes, and germs.

As we get older and nature's machinery slows down, this sloughing off of the dead skin becomes more desultory. We need help to restore the skin to a more youthful and vibrant appearance. That is where epidermabrasion with a Buf-Puf becomes invaluable. The Buf-Puf was invented by Dr. Norman Orentreich and is available at drug and cosmetics counters everywhere. Dr. Orentreich is my dermatological guru, and anything he does or recommends gets high marks in my book. His Buf-Puf is a textured cleansing sponge that gets rid of dead surface skin with its gentle abrasive action. I use it every other day with some cleansing lotion and get cleaning and epidermabrasion in one action. When my skin looks particularly dull, I increase the pressure and speed. I also use it in the shower or bath, particularly on the scaly areas of the elbows, knees, and feet. Since I started doing my own epidermabrasion, I haven't felt the need to do anything more radical as far as my complexion is concerned.

Dr. Orentreich believes that the skin of the average person over fifty needs rehabilitation in the form of what he terms "the three R's": replacing (minigraft or silicone), resurfacing (dermabrasion), or redraping (face-lift). When mere epidermabrasion and self-help are not enough, we should resort to one of the R's. Which one we choose should be determined by the nature of the problem.

REPLACEMENT. Wrinkles, furrows, "worry lines," pockmarks, and scars are the result of the loss of tissue, which causes the surface skin to collapse. The best way to eradicate these localized problems is by replacing the lost tissue. In the case of a deep or "ice-pick" scar, the solution is a minigraft. The scar is cut out of the skin with an instrument that might be described as a surgical hole-punch and replaced by a graft of normal skin from behind the ear.

The big problem for most of us is tiny wrinkles and furrows, "laugh lines" and "worry lines," the latter two aptly named, for in half a lifetime we've done a great deal of both. I've already mentioned that my problem was the tiny lines that had developed above my upper lip, which became even more pronounced in photographs. Of course, they could have been eradicated by skillful retouching, but I hate the look of a picture in which lines have been mechanically removed, leaving a masklike surface in which eyes and mouth leap out in bold relief.

I consulted Dr. Orentreich, and his suggestion was silicone shots. For years I'd heard about the bad effects of silicone injections, and I was more than a little skeptical about permitting the substance to be implanted in my face. There were so many horror stories: It could not be controlled; it moved around under the skin; it was toxic; it caused infection and ulceration.

Dr. Orentreich explained that the bad name had come from the use of massive injections of adulterated silicone for breast reconstruction. It was the uncontrolled shooting of an impure substance into fatty and glandular tissue by often unqualified individuals that caused the tragic results. What he proposed in my case was the use of droplets of medical-grade silicone, an unadulterated liquid substance prepared under sterile conditions and laboratory-tested. He had safely and successfully given silicone implants to hundreds of patients with far more serious conditions than mine. Although the doctor named no names, a little private investigation revealed that among them was what amounted to a hall of fame of fashion, theatrical, and social figures of both sexes.

A minute droplet of silicone was injected into each small wrinkle with the thinnest of needles. In time, my body's own collagen built up around the silicone, locking it in place. It has been several years since my last treatment, and there have been no ill effects and no recurrence of the problem.

It must be added that the FDA has never

approved silicone injections, nor has it made them illegal, although they are against the law in Nevada and cannot be used in California for breast implants. On the subject of breast re-sculpturing, medical-grade silicone enclosed in plastic sacks is currently being implanted safely and with no harmful aftermath.

The FDA has approved Zyderm, a bovine collagen derived from cowhides, for wrinkle and scar implantation. The safety and effectiveness of the product is unknown beyond a three-year period. Unlike silicone, there have been cases of allergic reactions. In addition, animal collagen is not as permanent as silicone; it is absorbed into the system rather than being held in place by the body's own collagen buildup around the implant.

RESURFACING. When you resurface the skin, you are literally peeling away the top layer and most of the afflictions contained in it. Almost all epidermal and some superficial dermal defects are removed. These include acne scars, pockmarks, age wrinkles, dark circles under the eyes, surface discoloration, warts, birthmarks, lesions, burn scars, precancerous black spots, and some skin cancers. For deep furrows and lines, silicone remains the best treatment. As our skins age, we probably will do best with a combination of resurfacing and replacement.

Some beauty institutions advertise that they do peeling. It is a very light peel, usually done by trained operators. It can't do any harm, but it can't do a great deal of good either, and I don't recommend it. This is a serious business and should be left in the hands of trained physicians and surgeons.

In my opinion, both the best and easiest method of resurfacing is *dermabrasion.* It is performed in a physician's office with a high-speed, rotating stainless-steel wire brush after the application of an ethyl chloride spray that freezes and anesthetizes the area. The upper layer of the skin is actually brushed off, and the whole face can be peeled in twenty minutes. The patient is usually ready to face the world in two weeks, although extremes of temperature, direct sunlight, and wind should be avoided for a month.

Chemosurgery is another method of resurfacing. It usually takes a stay of two or more days in the hospital and uses trichloroacetic acid to burn away the top layer of the skin. The results are striking and long-lasting, but it may be almost two months before the patient is ready to be seen in public. Alcohol, tobacco, and sunlight must be avoided for chemosurgery to be truly efficacious.

Cryotherapy is controlled burning by a freezing jet of gas, usually liquid nitrogen. It destroys the tissue by freezing it. In time, the epidermis forms a crust, which can be peeled off. The convalescence is swift, but the procedure may have to be done in a hospital, and repeated treatment is sometimes necessary.

REDRAPING. When there are sags and pouches, a complete or partial face-lift is the only solution. Before submitting to one, I would suggest obtaining several opinions. Find the plastic surgeon you really trust and try to see some examples of his work in the flesh rather than in photographs. There's nothing I distrust more than the before and after photographs one finds in books, magazines, and surgeons' offices. The "before" is usually wearing no makeup, has messy hair, and looks as if she just got up from a bad night's sleep and hasn't even washed her face yet. "After" has obviously been tarted up by the best cosmetician and hairdresser money can buy.

If you and your surgeon genuinely feel that everything is wrong, then the complete face-lift or rhytidectomy is the only solution. Usually, it is not necessary. Often, just doing the eyes (ble-pharoplasty) will do wonders. Removing those droops on the upper lid and sags on the lower lid can be enough to restore the well-rested and vital look that should be the only objective of plastic surgery. But this is delicate work and cannot be left to the local hack or quack. There is very little fatty tissue and there are many nerve endings in the skin around the eyes. A successful job will call upon all of the artistry of a skilled expert.

By way of resculpturing the features of the face and almost any part of the body, there is practically nothing that an excellent plastic surgeon cannot accomplish. The important word is *excellent.* Top reputations usually earn hefty fees, but one should never shop for bargains where one's face and body are concerned. Don't let anybody tell you these operations are snaps. They are dangerous, and the degree of risk is as high as the potential for lasting improvement in the quality of one's life. Before submitting to the knife, you must be aware that a plastic surgeon's mistakes are often irremediable, and the results can maim or disfigure you for life. I don't mean to sound negative. Plastic surgery is one of the great boons of modern times, but it should not be contemplated lightly. You really must know why you are doing it, the degree of competence of the surgeon, and whether it will truly solve the problems that are troubling you. You'll appreciate the new you only as well as you appreciated the old you. If everything works out in the affirmative, then go to it. When the time comes, if the motivations are right, I'll be more than happy to join you.

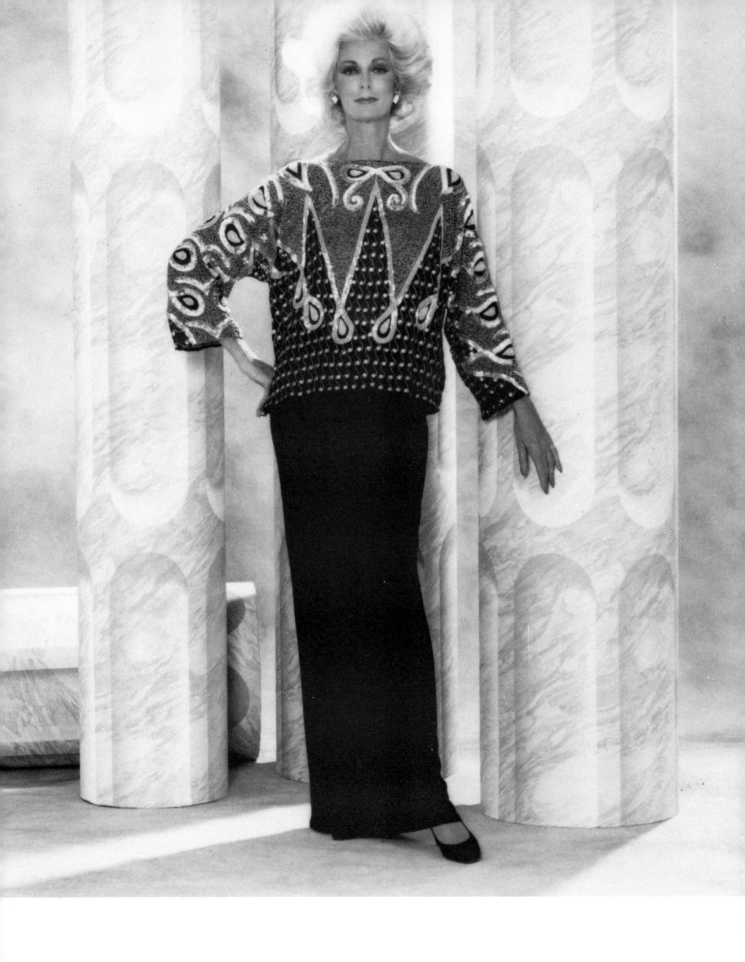

8

DRESSING

CLOTHES SHOULD NEVER
make the woman. The right dress is the one
enhanced by the woman wearing it. I'm not
really flattered when people only comment that
I'm wearing a fantastic dress. I'd much rather
hear them say it is a becoming dress, because
that implies that I look fantastic in it.

Everybody makes mistakes. I've got a closet
full of them. They are all beautiful and all completely wrong for me. I bought them because
they were the height of fashion. It was that old
bugaboo, "they." It was what "they" were
wearing that season, and I felt I had to have it,
although I should have known better. It was not
what *I* should have been wearing that season or
any other season. It was not right for my body,
my age, my style.

Sequin is a festive look—it's not for Sunday brunch. It's
not a necessity in one's wardrobe but can be a lovely
luxury if it suits your personality. (*Frank Maresca*)

We can't blame our mistakes on the designers. Designers are true to themselves, to their
image of what a line should be, which has to
change each season. It is not their fault that we
don't change each season but remain the same
people with the same individual stylistic needs.

Finding an individual style is one of the simplest things in the world. It depends on only
three things: the shape of the body, the coloring
of skin and hair, the life-style.

Let's go back to that three-way mirror and
have a good look. What are your assets? The
neck, the texture of the skin on the chest, the
shoulders, the length of the leg and shape of the
calf? Then those are the things your clothes
must display and enhance. What are your
liabilities? A thickening of the waist, a broad
beam, a fatty underarm? Those are the things to
be concealed and played down.

Any clothes that distort the body or emphasize its physical or aesthetic shortcomings are wrong. Personally, I'd like to put pants back on men. I'm too broad in the beam for them, and so are most of the women I know. Blue jeans should stay on the farm or on the very young. Designer jeans have to be one of the biggest fashion rip-offs of all time. Is it really worth all the extra money just to have some celebrity's or designer's name stamped on your fanny?

Nobody denies that throwing on a shirt and pants has a certain relaxed comfort, but if you're not going in for certain sports or physical labor, a shift is just as comfortable, and it covers a multitude of sins. A shift gives a flow of fabric. For most women my age, a long-sleeved shift is the best and simplest style. It can be dressed up with scarves and jewelry. In the evening, its Arabic cousin, the caftan, is timeless and extremely feminine.

There are exceptions. I know a woman who has very bad legs. It's a congenital thing—her mother had them and so do her sisters. She always thought of skirts as a kind of put-down. When pants came in, they were a blessing. Whatever happens in fashion, she should never give them up. She is a different person in them, more secure and at home with herself. Pants are her style, and fashion be damned!

Now, let's look at coloring. I have silver hair and an ivory skin. Nobody will ever talk me out of a bright red dress at any age. As our skin and hair pale, bright colors are marvelous. Any of the purples or lavenders are as bad on our bodies as they are on our faces. Green is bad on an olive complexion, and yellow is bad on a sallow one. As far as color is concerned, the skin is just another shade, but it is the most important one; every color we wear is the accessory and should be harmonious with it. It boils down to the basic fact that everything we put on our backs should accessorize us and not the reverse.

Once we've discovered our individual style, we can be ourselves. Away from the cameras,

I've discovered classic lines that hint at the lines of my body are best for me. I don't want a dress to advertise every secret asset or flaw. I'm also a paradox in clothes—the two things that suit me are the tailored look and the billowing romantic one. Both provide the illusion of perfection, and both are timeless. I save the romantic dresses for special occasions; my everyday look is always tailored.

Simplicity is the key to my individual style. It saves me a great deal of money, because there's such a wide range of ready-to-wear clothes that are both simple and well made. Seventh Avenue does them better than anybody in the world. Fashion gimmicks and froufrous are expensive. Only the highest-priced and most expert dressmakers know how to execute them so they don't look tawdry. When one adds the fact that there is only one season's wear out of them, I think they're out of the range of even my richest friends. Another good reason for timeless simplicity is that you don't see yourself coming and going in the latest fashion mandate. A lot of women find security in discovering three or four dresses just like the one they're wearing in the same room. The few times it has happened to me, I've got to admit it's only made me feel sadly lacking in imagination and individuality.

During the writing of this book, I've discovered that so many of the colorful and vivid places I remember so well no longer exist. What has happened to New York City is a metaphor for what I feel about clothes. All that had individual style in this city is falling victim to a uniform fashion for street after street of monolithic and boring glass boxes. We must not be like the city and fall victim to the newest fads of the fashion architects. That is what I call "todayism." Nothing becomes faded yesterday so quickly and inevitably as does today. When a woman reaches a certain point of wisdom about herself, fashion does not pass her by— she passes *it* by. She no longer permits fashion to lock her into chic boxes that momentarily glitter but are essentially as transparent and characterless as glass.

Oh, yes, I do occasionally indulge in the latest craze in makeup and clothes. I have not left all sense of fantasy behind in my childhood. But I always return to the tried and true, to what works best for me as an individual, and not only do I *not* consider myself a back number, but the people I know seem to think I'm an up-to-date and well-dressed woman. I love what's new and good. I can't stand what is only new and newer.

Style is timeless: It embraces the best of today and the promise of tomorrow without relinquishing the glories of yesterday.

For the last few years, I've been doing the catalogs for a shop called La Shack. The clothes are medium-priced ready-to-wear and similar to clothes that are available all over the country. I always find several things I want to own, because I know I'll get years of wear out of them. I've selected a few and would like to use them to illustrate everything I've been saying about style versus fashion.

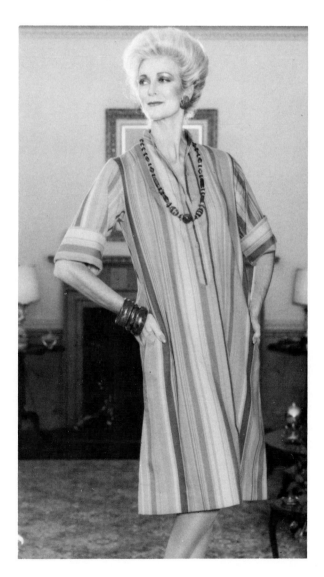

The shift. It is the staple of my wardrobe. You can dress it up or dress it down. You can work in the garden in it or wear it to a smart luncheon party. It covers a multitude of sins in a maximum of comfort. *(Frank Maresca)*

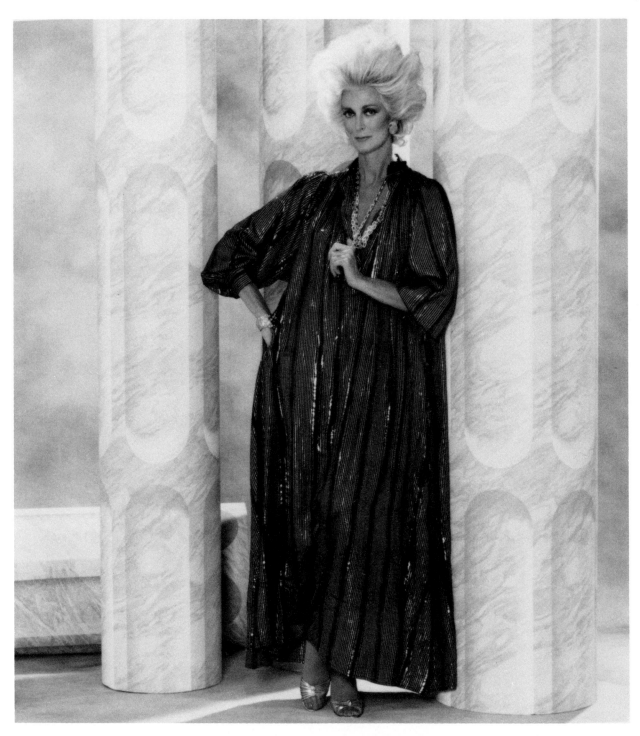

The caftan. (*Here and on facing page*): From the Arabian deserts comes the shift's glamorous evening cousin. Alluring in what it conceals, this timeless fashion can be worn to a dinner dance or for a romantic evening at home—the fabric dictates the use. In terry cloth, you can wear it poolside. In gold-threaded chiffon, you can wear it to a ball. (*Frank Maresca*)

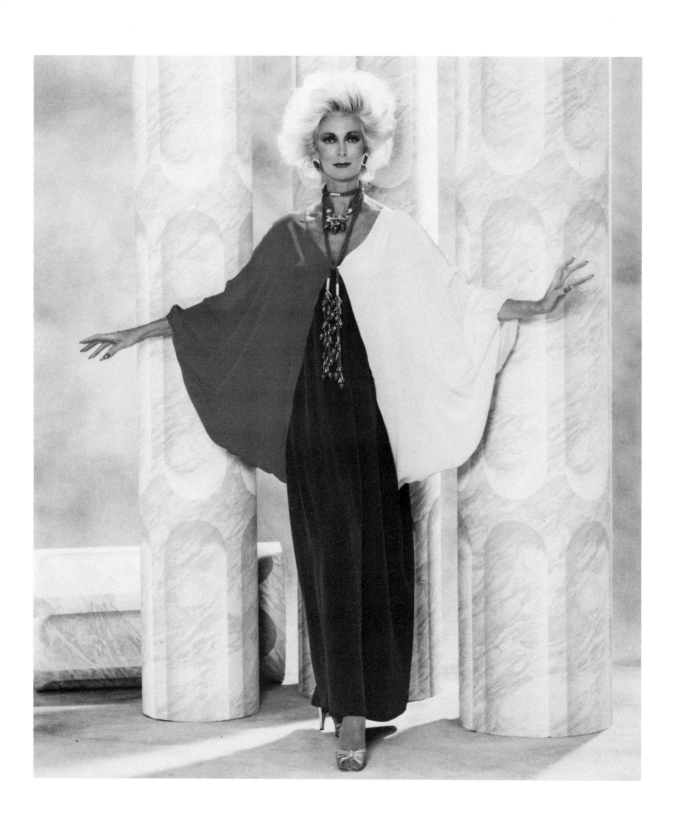

The knitted sweater is another classic and a lasting addition to any wardrobe. In glitter with a slimming evening skirt, you are ready for any formal evening function. In wool with a wool skirt, you're ready for all of your day-to-day activities, from office to PTA. In silk, it can take you through your entire day and right into the evening when you don't have time to change before the theater or a dinner party. (*Frank Maresca*)

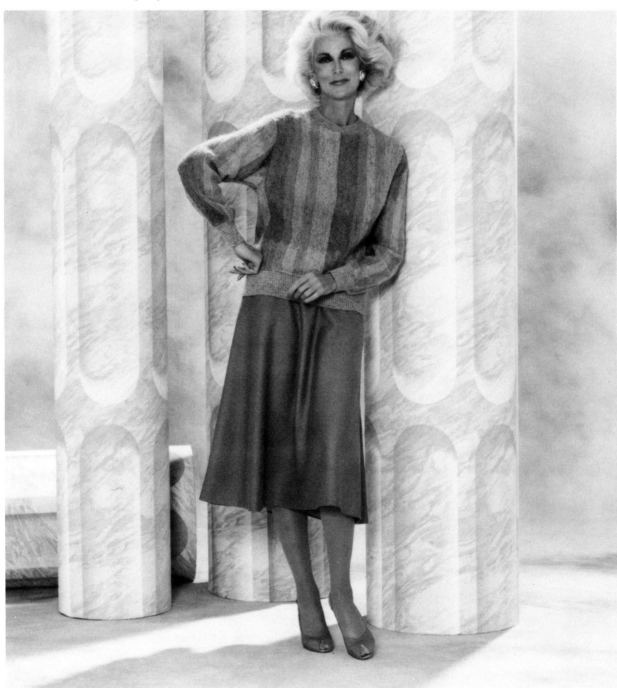

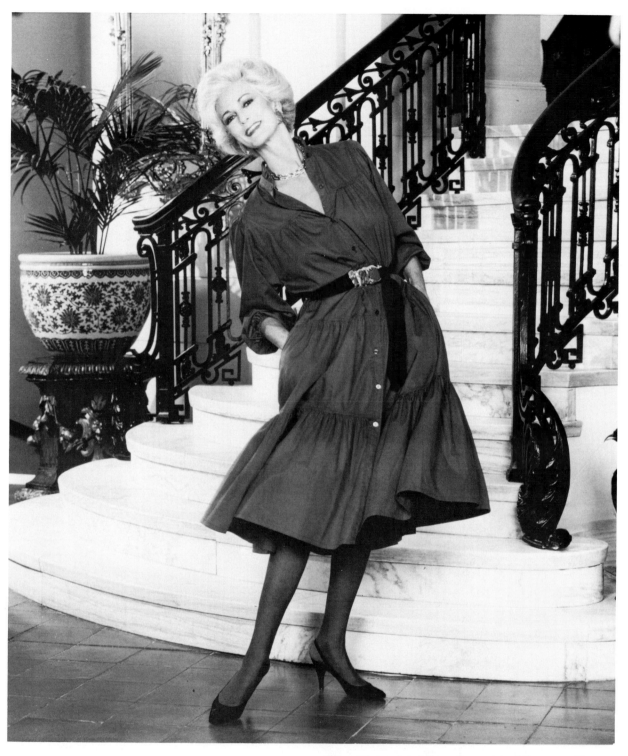

The shirtwaist defines the waist while concealing everything else. A timeless gem that is always in style no matter where fashion may be. Again, the fabric dictates its use. I've seen it in men's shirting and in silk satin, and it works as well in both. (*Frank Maresca*)

The halter top can be a gown or sundress, depending on length and fabric. The jersey number I'm wearing in this photo is one of my favorites. It hints at everything while actually revealing nothing. What's more, it packs like a dream. (*Frank Maresca*)

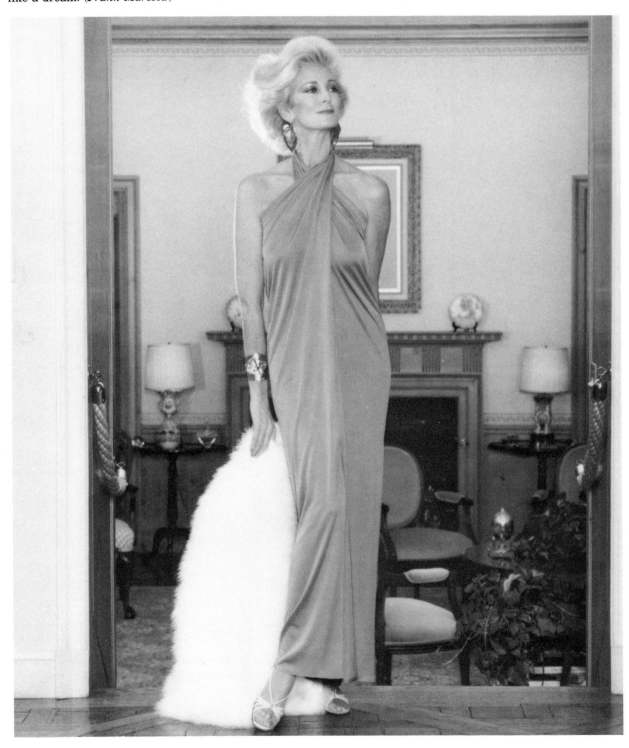

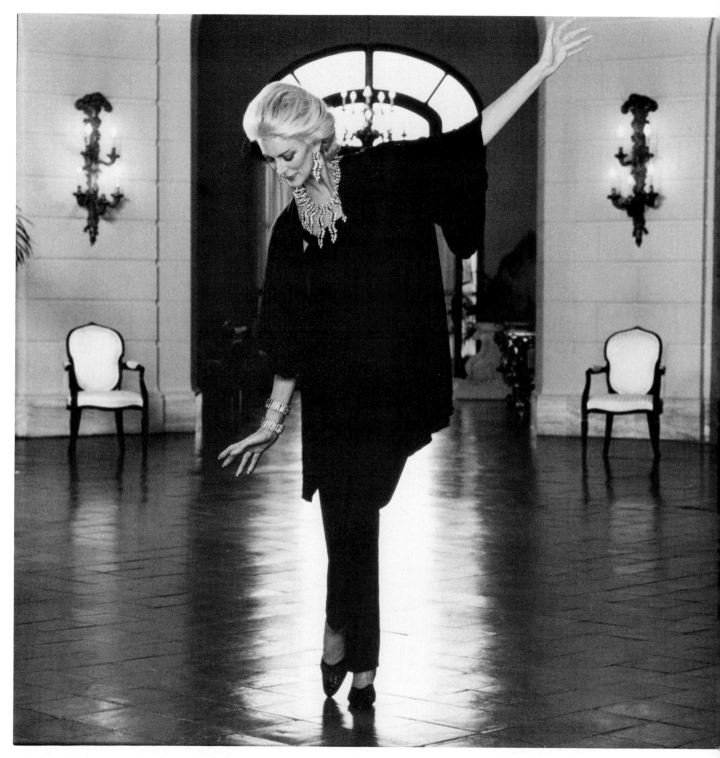

The "separates" look: Ideally, clothes should be made to fit the body rather than the body made to fit the clothes. Not many of us can, however, afford custom tailoring. The "separates" concept allows us to choose clothes that accommodate the changes in our bodies. The black three-piece silk outfit I'm wearing emphasizes the elegant yet not overdressed look. (*Frank Maresca*)

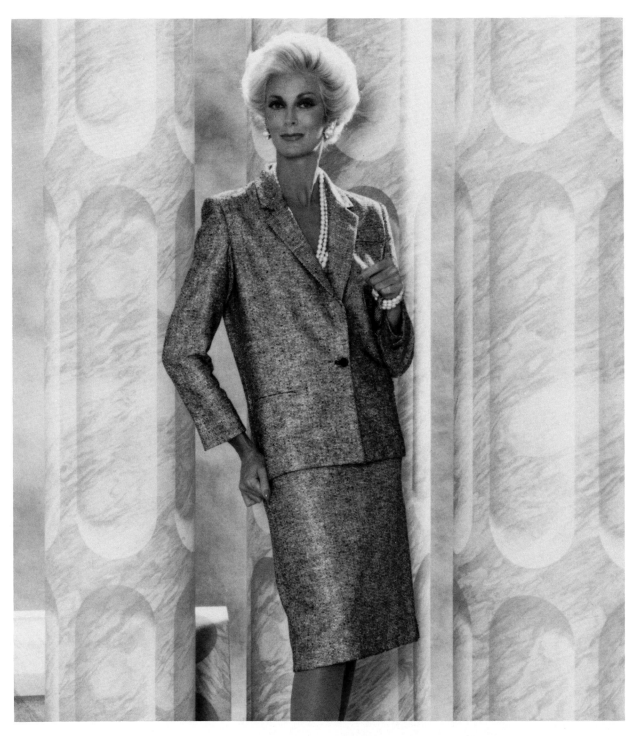

The tailored suit is never out of style. Whether you are too heavy, too thin, or just right, it will flatter your figure. In a gleaming heavy silk, it can serve for the dressiest occasions. In a nubby wool or tweed, it is the perfect fashion *"pour le sport."* In gray flannel, it is transformed into the businesswoman's uniform. (*Frank Maresca*)

The basic black dress, which speaks for itself. Never deride the idea of "the little black dress."
It works. (*Frank Maresca*)

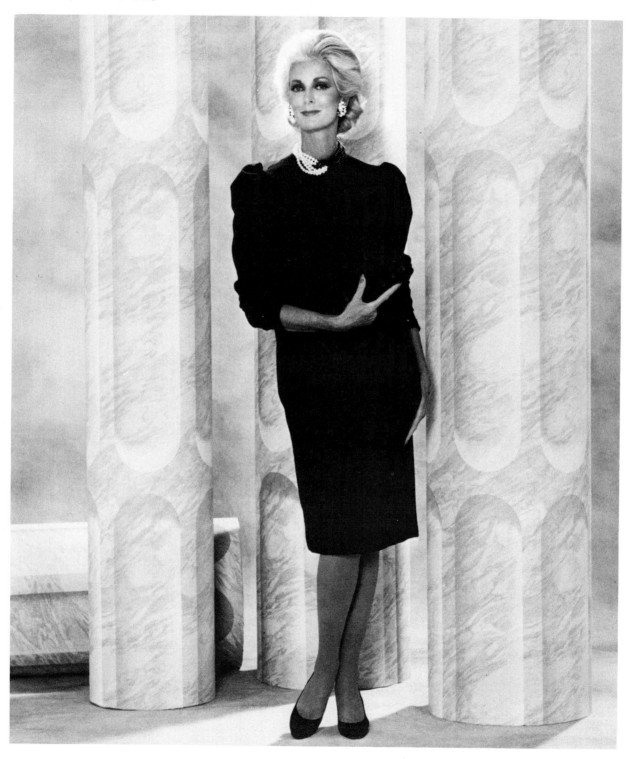

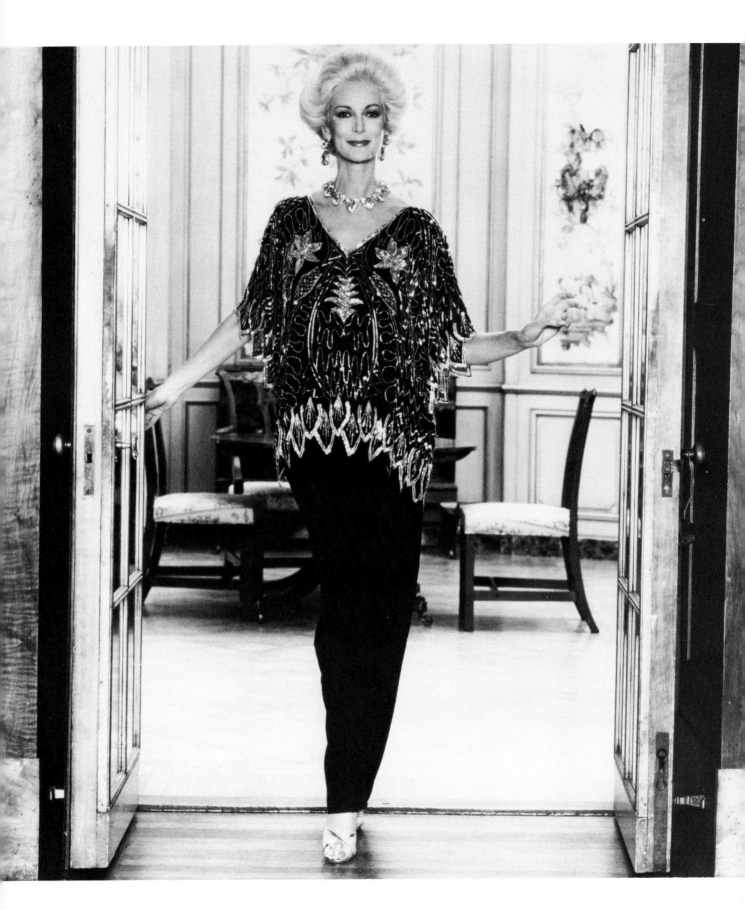

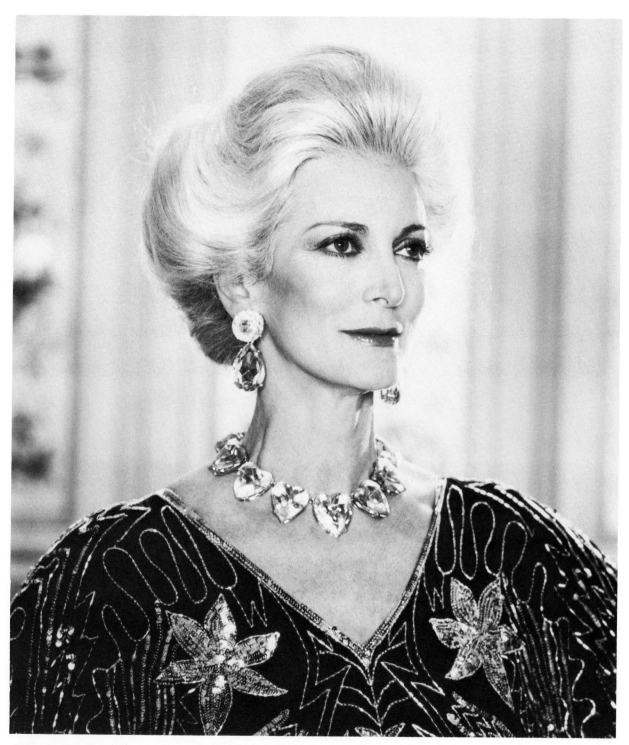

The sequinned look: a variation. What's important about handling sequins is not to overdo it. It can be a flattering and glamorous look if handled imaginatively. The evening top shown here (*facing page*) can be worn festively at home or, with accessories, to the theater or a gala evening out. Don't be afraid of bold accessories. (*Frank Maresca*)

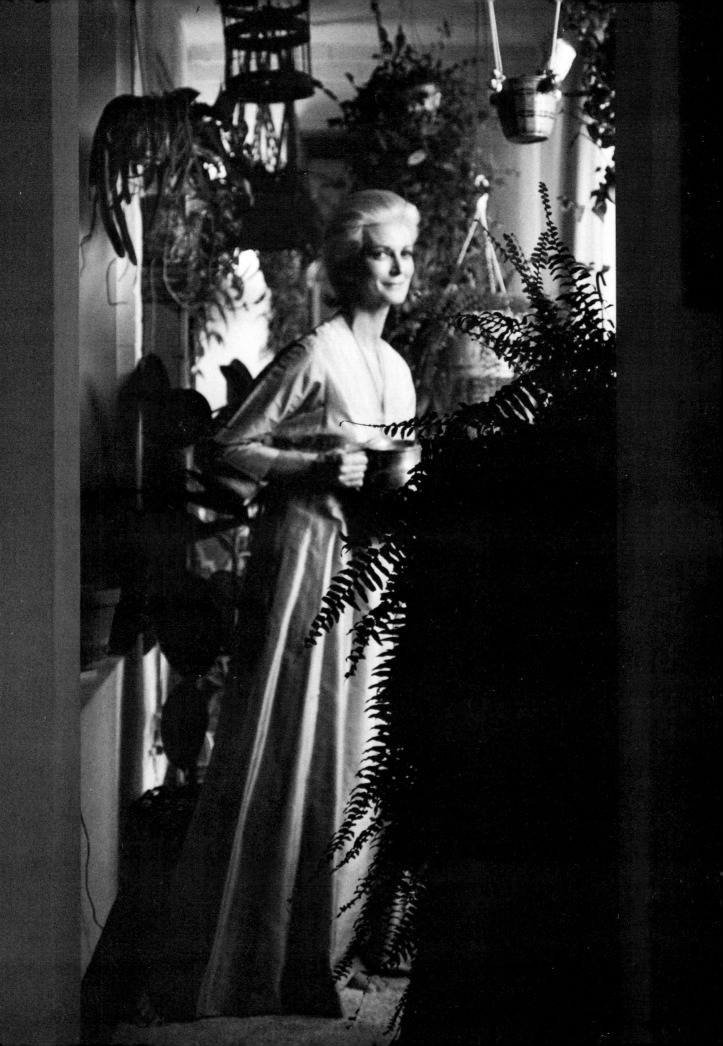

9

AT HOME WITH MYSELF

I LEARNED HOW TO BE AT home with myself when I discovered who I was, and that I liked the woman I had become. That can happen at any age. I was a late bloomer. I had been other people's fantasies for so long, it took a midlife crisis to shock me into being my own person. Being at home has nothing to do with where or how you live. In my time, I've inhabited many grand dwellings, and I now live in a four-room apartment. The difference between inhabiting and living in a place is enormous. You can live in a place and share it, or you can inhabit a place, and it makes no difference who else is there—you're only passing through.

To be at home is to see reflections of your life

and style in every corner. When you share your home, that sharing is part of the reflection. Allowing where you live to be somebody else's image of who you should be is dooming your real self to be forever passing through, for you will never find yourself in your surroundings.

My apartment is filled with souvenirs of my whole life. I look around and see pieces of my past and present and am never lonely in my home. I like being "at home" to my friends, entertaining and sharing where I live with those most meaningful to me. The place grew out of me. No decorator had a hand in it. It's a conglomeration of special bits and pieces going all the way back to Third Avenue and very unfashionable in any decorator's sense of the word. Things have come out of friends' attics, and storage, and old suitcases to find their places in my environment. The result is a mira-

My flourishing little greenhouse is a source of great satisfaction and joy.

cle to me, for it is everything I want in a home, a place where people can put their feet up and feel cozy and comfortable—I most of all.

I don't know if I'll ever marry or live with anybody again. It's no longer the most important thing in my life. If the right man came along, I'd be willing to give it a shot—but to be right, he would have to accept Carmen as she is and not as he fantasizes her; he'd have to take a hard look around my place and say, "I know this woman, and I like her." The bottom line is, I want to be liked as well as loved, just as I want to like as well as love the man I live with. Liking takes recognition and acceptance of all faults and virtues. Nothing else will do. If that happens, there is always room to absorb his souvenirs into my space. It would be the best of two worlds—his and mine.

At last, I'm at home with myself, and that suits me fine. It's my style.

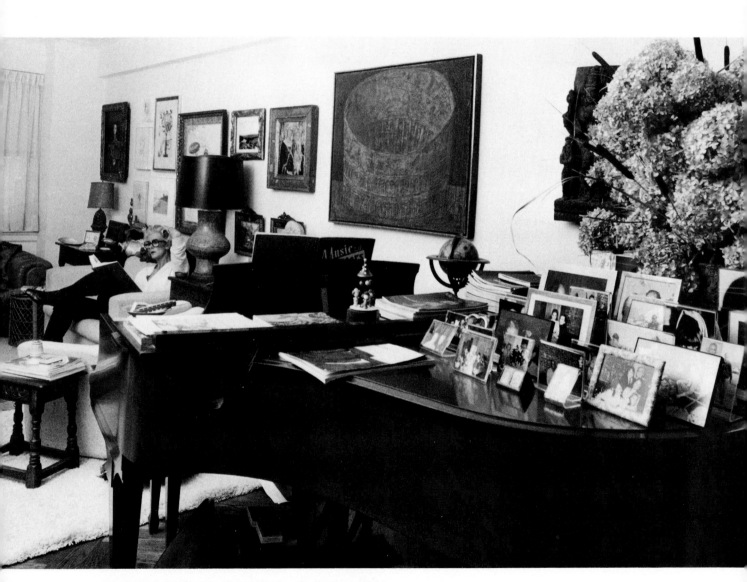

A piano cluttered with photographs of all those who mean the most in my life brings my world to me even in my most solitary moments.

196

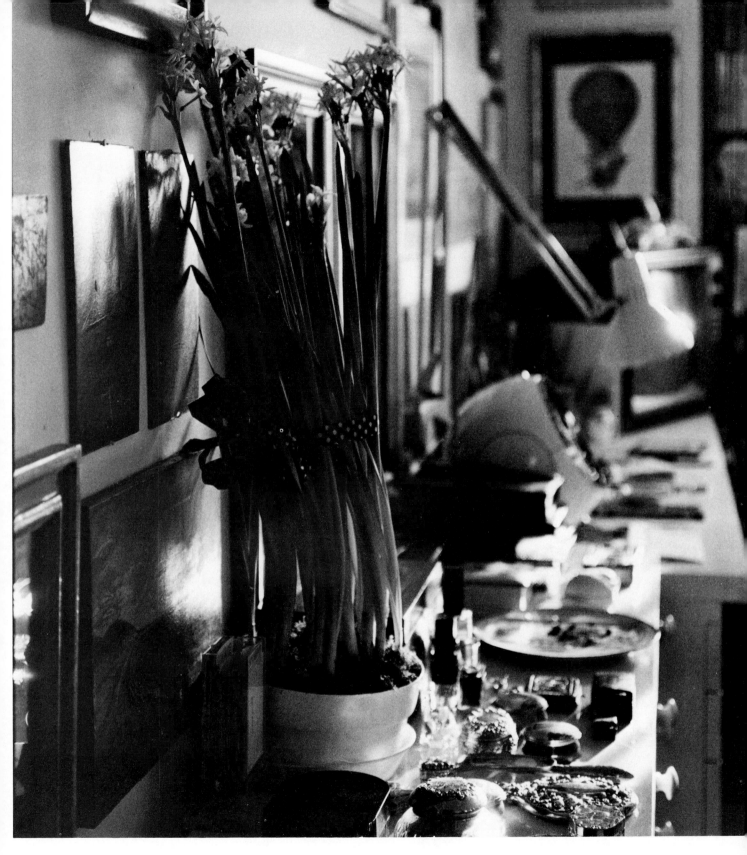

I love the orderly clutter of my bedroom, from books to television to souvenirs. I can bring a meal on a tray and find perfect contentment.

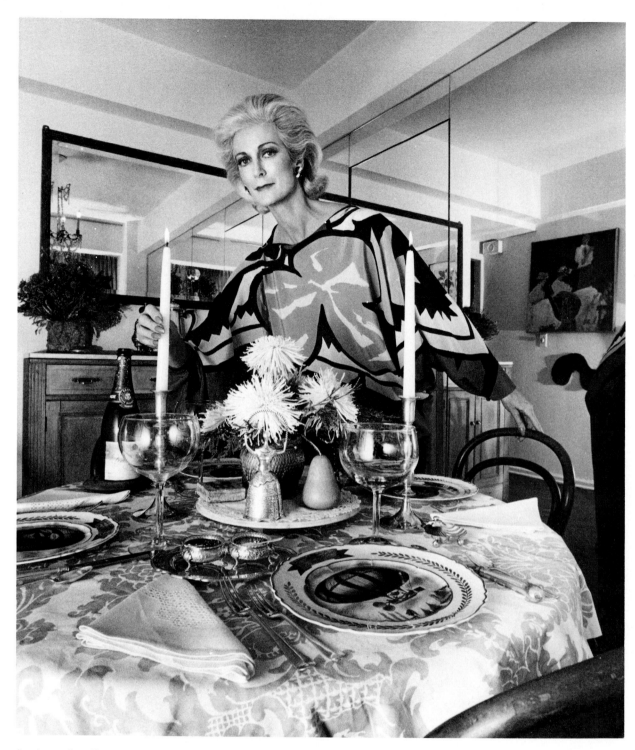

A mirrored wall makes my tiny dining room seem twice as large. I love to cook, set a pretty table, and dress up for an evening at home with good friends. The dress was designed by my good friend Michael Vollbracht. I adore his combinations of classic line and daring original prints.

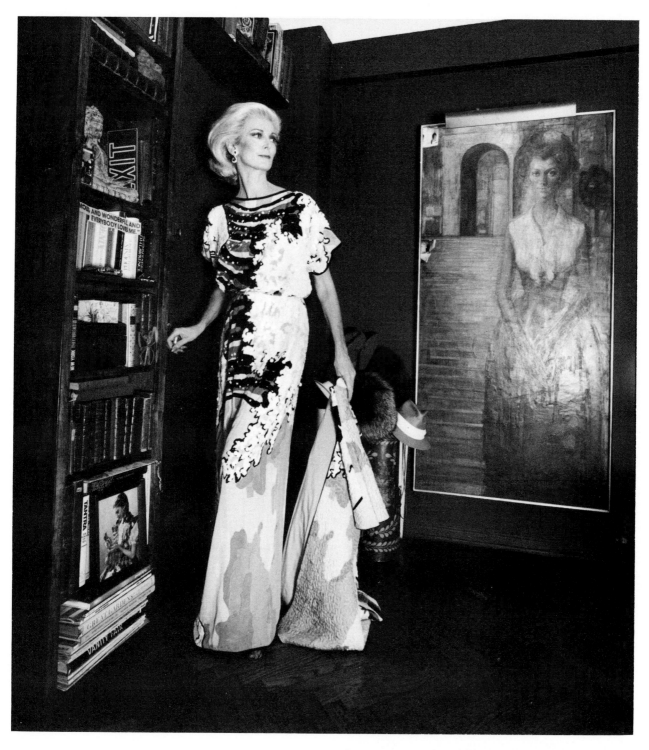

On my way to a big night on the town. As you can see, my small foyer doubles as a library. Again, I'm wearing a Vollbracht. This time, the print is picked out in glitter and has a matching wrap. Large women should never be afraid of big, bold prints that make dramatic statements.

INDEX

202